Clinical Pharmacology
and Practical Prescribing
on the move

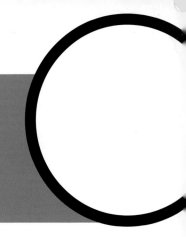

Clinical Pharmacology
and Practical Prescribing
on the move

Authors: **James Turnbull**
and Matthew Tate
Editorial Advisor: **Peter Jackson**

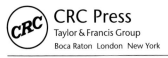

CRC Press
Taylor & Francis Group
Boca Raton London New York

CRC Press is an imprint of the
Taylor & Francis Group, an **informa** business

CRC Press
Taylor & Francis Group
6000 Broken Sound Parkway NW, Suite 300
Boca Raton, FL 33487-2742

© 2016 by Taylor & Francis Group, LLC
CRC Press is an imprint of Taylor & Francis Group, an Informa business

No claim to original U.S. Government works

Printed and bound in India by Replika Press Pvt. Ltd.

Printed on acid-free paper
Version Date: 20150417

International Standard Book Number-13: 978-1-4441-7603-2 (Pack - Book and Ebook)

Library of Congress Cataloging-in-Publication Data

Turnbull, James, 1979- , author.
    Clinical pharmacology and practical prescribing on the move / James Turnbull, Matthew Tate.
    p. ; cm. -- (Medicine on the move)
    Includes bibliographical references and index.
    ISBN 978-1-4441-7603-2 (hardcover : alk. paper)
    I. Tate, Matthew, 1987- , author. II. Title. III. Series: Medicine on the move (CRC Press)
    [DNLM: 1. Pharmacology, Clinical--Examination Questions. 2. Pharmacology, Clinical--Outlines. 3. Drug Prescriptions--Examination Questions. 4. Drug Prescriptions--Outlines. 5. Pharmaceutical Preparations--Examination Questions. 6. Pharmaceutical Preparations--Outlines. QV 18.2]

    RS57
    615.1--dc23
    2015014386

Visit the Taylor & Francis Web site at
http://www.taylorandfrancis.com

and the CRC Press Web site at
http://www.crcpress.com

Contents

Preface

Have you ever found pharmacology overwhelmingly complicated? Are you daunted by the prospect of prescribing? Or are you simply short of time and have exams looming? If so, this practical guide will help you. Written by doctors for doctors, this book presents information in a wide range of formats including flow charts, boxes, summary tables and diagrams.

Pharmacology and the prescription of medicines are fascinating topics and ubiquitous within medicine, yet many junior doctors feel unprepared when they start work, both with their underlying knowledge of pharmacology and with the practicalities of prescribing.

It can seem challenging to gain the information needed to practise medical prescribing safely and effectively using the plethora of sources available. Many focus on basic pharmacology, often providing more information than is required for the busy doctor. Others focus solely on prescribing. The *British National Formulary* is an excellent resource, but due to its inclusiveness, lack of pharmacology and constraints based upon drug licensing, it cannot always provide the information needed for day-to-day work.

In writing this book we have drawn upon our personal experiences, one of us as a former clinical pharmacist, and both as junior doctors, to provide an appropriate degree of working pharmacological knowledge and practical prescribing advice and to complement other reference sources. We also aim to assist those who will be sitting the Prescribing Skills Assessment (PSA).

The book is divided into three parts: clinical pharmacology (background knowledge for working practice), drugs and practical prescribing (class based pharmacology and drug information) and self-assessment (a guide to the upcoming Prescribing Skills Assessment [PSA]).

In Part II, Drugs and Practical Prescribing, each drug class has been reviewed to highlight the key issues commonly faced by the junior doctor. Accordingly, the depth of coverage in this section varies between chapters and each drug class. Cross-references between chapters are available to aid understanding by relating the topic to more detailed or associated content.

We are taught in medicine that 'common things are common', and following that theme, this book does not aim to provide exhaustive lists. Any dosing, adverse effects or interactions quoted focus on the common and the important, and do not necessarily cover the full range of indications or effects. You will find more information presented on the drugs that in our experience you will likely encounter more frequently. The exception to the 'common' rule is where significant risks are associated with less common drugs; these are dealt with in more detail.

Where complex prescribing regimens are discussed, this book explains the rationale of each and provides example prescriptions. However, please be aware that it is common practice for guidelines to be produced locally and we would always recommend that readers use these documents preferentially.

We hope this book will offer clinicians a portable and practical guide to prescribing that will complement larger reference texts. We hope you find it helpful!

AUTHORS

Dr James Turnbull MPharm ClinDip Pharm MBChB Hons - Specialist Registrar in Anaesthesia, Health Education Yorkshire and the Humber, UK
Dr Matthew Tate MBChB (Hons) DTM&H, Core Medical trainee 2, The Hillingdon Hospitals NHS Foundation Trust, London, UK

EDITORIAL ADVISOR

Peter R. Jackson MBChB, PhD, FRCP, Consultant Physician and Honorary Reader in Clinical Pharmacology & Therapeutics, Royal Hallamshire Hospital, Sheffield, UK

EDITOR-IN-CHIEF

Rory Mackinnon BSc(Hons) MBChB MRCGP GP Partner, Dr Cloak & Partners, Southwick Health Centre, Sunderland, UK

SERIES EDITORS

Sally Keat MBChB BMedSci MRCP Core Medical Trainee Year 2 in Barts Health NHS Trust
Thomas Locke BSc, MBChB, DTM&H, MRCP(UK) Core Medical Trainee Year 2, Northwick Park Hospital, London Northwest Healthcare, London, UK
Andrew MN Walker BMedSci MBChB MRCP (London) British Heart Foundation Clinical Research Fellow and Honorary Specialist Registrar in Cardiology, University of Leeds, UK

Acknowledgements

The authors would like to thank the following people for their contribution towards the production of this book:

- Dr Peter Jackson – for services above and beyond the call of duty
- Dr Christopher Turnbull – for his general help and counsel, in addition to editing duties
- Sheffield Teaching Hospital and Broadsword UK Limited – for allowing use of the drug charts in the book
- My more than patient family: Janine, Alex, Jake and Esme

List of abbreviations

DRUG DOSING AND ROUTES OF ADMINISTRATION

- OD: once daily
- BD: twice daily
- TDS: three times daily
- QDS: four times daily
- ON: at night
- Nocte: at night
- Mane: in the morning
- q4–6h: every 4–6 hours
- PO: orally
- PR: rectally
- IV: intravenous
- IM: intramuscular
- SC: subcutaneous
- NG: nasogastric

ABBREVIATIONS

- 5-ASA: 5 aminosalicylic acid (mesalazine)
- 5-HT: serotonin
- ACE inhibitors: angiotensin converting enzyme inhibitors
- ACh: acetylcholine
- ADH: anti-diuretic hormone
- ATPase: adenosine triphosphatase
- AV: atrioventricular
- BG: blood glucose
- BNF: British National Formulary
- *C. diff*: *Clostridium difficile*
- Ca^{2+}: Calcium ion
- CAP: community acquired pneumonia
- CCF: congestive cardiac failure
- CD: Crohn's disease
- Cl^-: Chloride ion
- CNS: central nervous system
- COPD: chronic obstructive pulmonary disease
- COX: cyclooxygenase
- CSF: cerebrospinal fluid
- CYP450: Cytochrome P450
- DKA: Diabetic ketoacidosis

- DPI: dry powder inhaler
- DVT: deep vein thrombosis
- EC: enteric coated
- ECT: electro-convulsive therapy
- ED: Emergency Department
- ENT: ear, nose and throat
- GABA: gamma-aminobutyric acid
- GI: gastrointestinal
- GORD: gastro-oesophageal reflux disease
- GTN: glyceryl trinitrate
- HAP: hospital acquired pneumonia
- HIT: heparin induced thrombocytopaenia
- HIV: human immunodeficiency virus
- IBD: inflammatory bowel disease
- INR: international normalised ratio
- K^+: Potassium ion
- L-dopa: levodopa
- LFT: liver function test
- LMWH: low molecular weight heparin
- LRTI: lower respiratory tract infection
- MAOI: monoamine oxidase inhibitor
- MDI: metered dose inhaler
- MR (m/r): modified release (analogous to slow release)
- MRSA: methicillin resistant *Staphylococcus aureus*
- Na^+: Sodium ion
- NAPQI: *N*—acetyl-*p*-benzoquinone imine (toxic paracetamol metabolite)
- NICE: The National Institute for Health and Care Excellence
- NMJ: neuromuscular junction
- NMS: neuroleptic malignant syndrome
- NSAIDs: non-steroidal anti-inflammatory drugs
- OA: osteoarthritis
- PCI: percutaneous coronary intervention
- PDE: phosphodiesterase
- PE: pulmonary embolus
- PPI: proton pump inhibitor
- PT: prothrombin time
- PTH: parathyroid hormone
- PVD: peripheral vascular disease
- RA: rheumatoid arthritis
- SIADH: syndrome of inappropriate anti-diuretic hormone secretion
- SJS: Stevens Johnson syndrome
- SLE: systemic lupus erythematosus
- SR: slow release (analogous to modified release)

- SSRI: selective serotonin reuptake inhibitor
- $t_{1/2}$: half-life
- TB: tuberculosis
- TDM: therapeutic drug monitoring
- TEN: toxic epidermal necrolysis
- TPN: total parenteral nutrition
- TSH: thyroid stimulating hormone
- UC: ulcerative colitis
- Vd: volume of distribution
- VTE: venous thromboembolism

An explanation of the text

The book is divided into three parts: clinical pharmacology, drugs and practical prescribing, and a self-assessment section. We have used bullet points to keep the text concise and supplemented this with a range of diagrams, pictures and MICRO-boxes (explained below).

Where possible we have included treatment options for the conditions covered. Nevertheless, drug sensitivities and clinical practices are constantly under review, so always check your local guidelines for up-to-date information.

You will find the following resources useful for additional information about any of the drugs mentioned in this book:

BNF (at http://www.bnf.org/bnf/index.htm)

eMC (at http://www.medicines.org.uk/emc/)

MICRO-facts

These boxes expand on the text and contain clinically relevant facts and memorable summaries of the essential information.

MICRO-print

These boxes contain additional information to the text that may interest certain readers but is not essential for everybody to learn.

MICRO-case

These boxes contain clinical cases relevant to the text and include a number of summary bullet points to highlight the key learning objectives.

MICRO-references

These boxes contain references to important clinical research and national guidance.

MICRO-monitoring

These boxes contain information on therapeutic drug monitoring (TDM) for drugs where monitoring plasma levels is part of clinical practice.

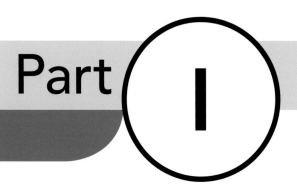

Part I

Clinical pharmacology

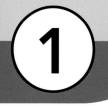

1 Clinical pharmacokinetics

Pharmacokinetics can be considered the aspect of pharmacology concerned with 'what the body does to the drug'. This aspect of pharmacology and the factors discussed below are relevant to how drugs are administered, dealt with by the body and finally eliminated.

1.1 BASIC PRINCIPLES OF PHARMACOKINETICS

DRUG CONCENTRATION/TIME CURVE

- This is the foundation of pharmacokinetics and all of the factors discussed below relate to this concept (Fig. 1.1).
  - After a drug reaches the blood stream it starts to distribute throughout the body, and actually starts to be eliminated.
  - For orally administered drugs there is also an absorption phase as the drug passes into the circulation.
  - a to b oral absorption takes place.
  - Point b: Peak serum drug concentration in the plasma.
  - Point b to c (α phase):
    - Drug distribution within the tissues occurs simultaneously with elimination, removing drug from the plasma more rapidly compared with elimination alone.
    - The duration of this phase depends upon how much the drug exists outside the plasma in equilibrium (Vd, see below), and how rapid the distribution is.
  - Point c to d (β phase):
    - Where reduction in plasma drug concentration is due mainly to elimination.

> ## MICRO-facts
> Most modified release preparations artificially alter the apparent drug concentration/time curve by slowly releasing the drug. This reduces the maximal concentration, but maintains higher levels for longer. See Fig. 1.2.

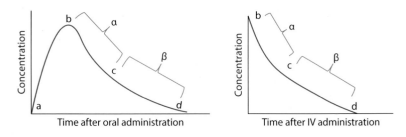

Fig. 1.1 Drug concentration/time curve.

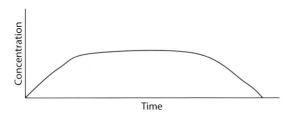

Fig. 1.2 Drug concentration/time curve for modified release preparations.

BIOAVAILABILITY

- This is the amount of drug that passes into the plasma after oral administration.
- By definition, the bioavailability of an IV preparation is 100%.
- Bioavailability is affected by the ability of the intestines to absorb the drug and by the extent of 'first pass metabolism':
  - Absorption
    - Non-ionized (lipid soluble/lipophilic) drugs are more readily absorbed as they pass through the lipid bilayer of the cell walls of the small intestine.
    - Environmental factors and physiochemical interactions are also implicated, and in clinical practice must be considered.
      - Food: many medications (e.g. oral penicillin) are subject to considerable decreased absorption if given with food.
      - Chelation/binding: drugs such as tetracyclines are chelated (chemically bound) if administered with metal ions (e.g. ferrous sulphate). Cholestyramine also binds many drugs, reducing absorption if it is co-administered.
  - 'First pass metabolism'
    - Any drug administered orally is absorbed through the bowel wall into the hepatic portal vein and subsequently to the liver.

- If significant liver metabolism deactivates the drug at this stage, limited quantities of active drug will be delivered to the systemic circulation.
- For this reason many drugs cannot be effectively administered orally and routes bypassing the liver (e.g. sublingual, rectal, transcutaneous or via injection) are used instead.
- Examples include **glyceryl trinitrate** and **fentanyl**.

MICRO-print

- Bioavailability varies enormously between drugs.
- Only 0.64% of the orally administered dose of **Alendronate** passes into the systemic circulation (similar low bioavailability is seen with all bisphosphonates).
- **Ciprofloxacin's** bioavailability is around 80% meaning I.V. preparations are only needed in those for whom oral administration is unsuitable.
- The first pass effect may be used for clinical effect. For example, 'pro-drugs' where an inactive metabolite is given which undergoes first pass metabolism to become the active drug. An example is codeine which is converted to morphine and other active compounds.

HALF-LIFE ($t_{1/2}$)

- Time taken for the amount of drug in the body or plasma to decrease by one half.
- For example, if there is 10 mg/L of drug in the plasma, and 24 hours later there is only 5 mg/L, the half-life is said to be 24 hours.
- Drugs with a long half-life exist largely outside the plasma (i.e. high Vd).
- This increases time to steady state (see below) and increases the time taken for drugs to be eliminated from the body.

MICRO-facts

For a drug with a long half-life the clinical effect will persist for some time, even after the patient has stopped taking it. You must take this into account when clinically assessing the patient or prescribing other medication. For example, the half-life of amiodarone is very long and the drug has multiple interactions.

- Drugs with a short half-life may have rapid effects due to a small Vd (see below) but the effect will wear off quickly.
- These drugs will often need repeated injections or be administered as a constant infusion.

Clinical pharmacology

MICRO-facts

- Clinicians must be aware of medications with a short half-life that are being used to influence a drug with a long half-life; for example, using naloxone to reverse an opioid overdose.
- Most opioids have a longer $t_{1/2}$ than naloxone, meaning the patient will initially improve but will exhibit signs of overdose again if the naloxone effect wears off before the opioid. A naloxone infusion may be appropriate in this scenario.

STEADY STATE (SS)

- If a drug is administered regularly and before the previous dose has been eliminated from the plasma, then the plasma concentration of the drug will build up (as will the tissue concentrations if the drug distributes outside of the plasma).
- This process will continue until a dynamic equilibrium is reached between administration and elimination, the 'steady state' (see Fig. 1.3).
- This usually occurs after 4 to 5 half-lives of the drug.
- If a drug given daily has a very short half-life then this accumulation will not occur as elimination will outpace the rate of administration.
- Steady state is particularly important for drugs with half-lives longer than 24 hours, as daily administration of the drug will lead to accumulation.

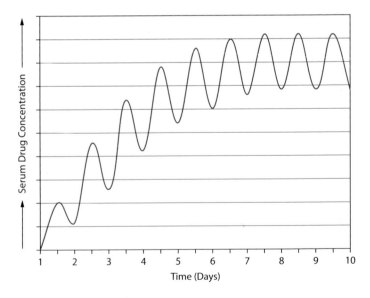

Fig. 1.3 Steady-state example of an orally administered drug.

> ### MICRO-facts
> Whether you are using clinical parameters (e.g. blood pressure) or drug levels to show efficacy always question whether the levels reached steady state (i.e. is this medication working to its full effect?). This will affect your assessment of whether further medication is required.

THE APPARENT 'VOLUME OF DISTRIBUTION' (Vd)

- Vd simply quantifies the distribution of a drug between the plasma and the rest of the body and is usually measured in L.
  - May be adapted and expressed as L/kg body weight.
- The numbers produced by calculation of Vd are purely conceptual. Vd = total amount of drug in body (mg)/plasma concentration (mg/L)
- Therefore drugs that have high plasma levels (e.g. highly bound to plasma proteins) are said to have a 'low volume of distribution'.
- Whereas those which exist largely outside the plasma, such as lipophilic (fat soluble) drugs are said to have a 'high volume of distribution'.
- This will influence the half-life of the drug as a high Vd will effectively create a 'store' of drug in the tissues that will take longer to return to the plasma and be eliminated (i.e. the half-life is prolonged).

Compartment models

- As implied by the volume of distribution model, drugs can exist outside of the plasma and be distributed into other tissues or 'compartments'. Examples include:
  - Fat tissue
  - Intracellular fluid
  - Extracellular fluids
    - Blood plasma
    - Interstitial fluid
    - Transcellular fluid (the 'third space' e.g. pleural space or CSF)
- Distribution into these compartments is dependent on many physical properties of the drug such as charge, solubility and protein binding in the plasma.
- Distribution is driven by concentration towards a dynamic equilibrium. The time it takes to occur represents the α phase of the drug concentration/time curve.
- Any change in concentration in one of the compartments will lead to redistribution from the others to maintain this equilibrium.
- The majority of drugs are only excreted from the plasma compartment (e.g. by glomerular filtration). Therefore, complete removal of a drug from

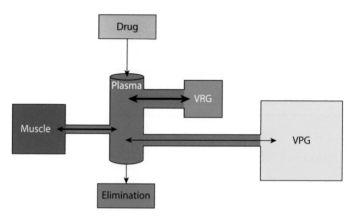

Fig. 1.4 The compartment model (basic three compartment model). Here size of the boxes represents compartment distribution volume, and width of arrows represents relative cardiac output.

the body will require multiple repetitions of redistribution from other body compartments to the plasma. For some drugs this process takes a considerable time, and for example, is the reason why amiodarone has such a long half-life and requires large loading doses. This process is outlined in Fig. 1.4.

- After administration, drug not eliminated from the plasma will be subject to distribution.
- Distribution into the tissues depends upon the relative cardiac output received and propensity of drug to distribute into that tissue.
- Initially the highest concentration of drug will be exposed to the vessel rich groups (VRG, e.g. brain, heart, kidneys) due to high cardiac output to these areas.
- Subsequently any further drug not eliminated will be exposed to the other groups with poorer blood supply but higher storage capacity (e.g. muscle, followed by the vessel poor group [VPG] such as adipose tissue).
- Lipophilic drugs (e.g. fentanyl) are highly distributed. Initially they move rapidly out of the plasma and into the VRG. Subsequently they are redistributed into the large capacity adipose tissue. Due to the lipophilic nature of these drugs, they are more slowly distributed back into the plasma for elimination thus extending the half-life.

LINEAR AND NON-LINEAR PHARMACOKINETICS

- These factors relate to the steady-state plasma concentrations which will be achieved following drug administration and subsequent elimination.
- As such they are important considerations when considering maintenance doses (see Ch. 2, Section 2.3).

Clinical pharmacology

Linear (first order) kinetics

- For the majority of drugs in clinical use, a higher plasma concentration results in a faster rate of elimination (i.e. elimination is proportional to concentration).
- At steady state, a linear relationship is established between drug concentration and the daily dose administered.
- In clinical practice this relationship has two principal effects:
  - Provides a linear and predictable response to dose change (stage a in Fig. 1.5). In this case doubling the daily dose will double the plasma level.
  - Provides concentration-dependent elimination.
    - Half-life remains constant throughout elimination stage (as seen in Fig. 1.6).
- This proportionality is known as 'First Order' kinetics.

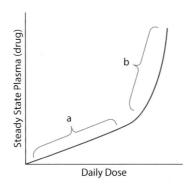

Fig. 1.5 Steady-state plasma concentration and daily dose. (a) Linear 'first order' response: A change in dose is associated with a proportional increase in steady-state plasma concentration. (b) Non-linear 'zero order' response: between stage a and b there is a rapid and progressive increase in steady-state plasma concentration as the dose increases representing saturation of metabolism/elimination pathways.

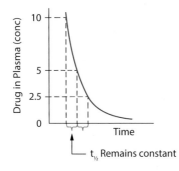

Fig. 1.6 First order drug elimination from the plasma. Note that the half-life is constant.

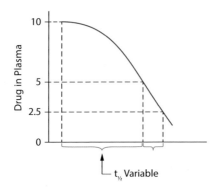

Fig. 1.7 Zero order drug elimination from the plasma. Variable half-life indicated.

Non-linear (zero order) kinetics

- If the metabolic or excretory pathways become saturated then giving a higher dose will not lead to an increase in elimination – this is called non-linear (zero order) kinetics.
- At this point further increases in dose will lead to a disproportionate accumulation of drug and significant rise in plasma concentration (see Fig. 1.5).
- Zero order kinetics also affects the elimination of drug from the body (Fig. 1.7).
  - The non-linear rate is due to initial slow elimination which accelerates as the plasma concentration falls.
  - This non-linearity means the half-life is not constant and varies with the plasma concentration. This reduces predictability of dose changes and plasma concentration.
- Clinically this means a small increase in dose may lead to large and potentially toxic plasma levels.

Zero order kinetics

- All drugs would undergo non-linear pharmacokinetics if they were given in doses high enough to saturate their metabolism/excretory pathways.
- The only drug for which this is seen commonly is phenytoin, however this is also the case for ethanol.
- After alcohol (ethanol) consumption, the calculation of the units left in the bloodstream is often said to be worked out by removing one unit per hour (representing maximum elimination capacity), which is why it may not be safe to drive the morning after a heavy night!

2 Clinical application of pharmacokinetics

2.1 PRINCIPLES OF DOSING

- The ultimate aim of drug dosing is to administer sufficient drug to produce a desired clinical effect but without inducing toxicity.
- Neither peak serum or trough concentrations should dip out of range (Fig. 2.1).
- Dosing regimens are predominantly dictated by the duration of action of the drug or its active metabolites, i.e. the respective half-lives.
- Half-lives of drugs can vary from minutes (e.g. remifentanil) to months (e.g. amiodarone).
- In this respect short acting drugs can be considered to be those eliminated within a normal dosing period (i.e. 24 hours). This would usually indicate a half-life of less than 5 hours.
- With short acting drugs (short half-life) there are four ways to ensure efficacy between doses:
    1. Administer a large dose (only if high peak serum levels don't result in toxicity).
    2. Administer multiple doses (dividing doses reduces peak levels).
    3. Administer a modified release preparation.
    4. Administer via constant IV infusion.
- Different considerations are required for long acting drugs (long half-life).
    - If drugs are not eliminated from the body before the next dose is administered, accumulation will occur until steady state.
    - Where clinical efficacy of the drug is found only after reaching steady state concentrations (after 4 to 5 $t_{1/2}$), there will be a delay between starting treatment and clinical effect.
    - However, this delay may not be clinically acceptable, for example a patient needing chemical cardioversion with amiodarone.
- In these cases therapy is often initiated using loading doses, and then followed with a maintenance regimen as discussed below.

2.2 LOADING DOSES

- Loading doses are simply a 'booster' dose to get plasma concentrations to an effective level.

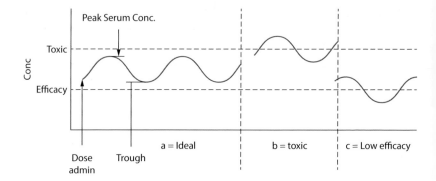

Fig. 2.1 Intermittent drug administration and drug concentration variance.

- Drugs with a short $t_{1/2}$ will often achieve efficacy with the 'normal dose' due to limited distribution (low Vd) therefore a 'loading dose' is not required.
- Drugs with a long $t_{1/2}$ may take a considerable time for plasma levels to reach therapeutic levels due to extensive distribution outside the plasma (high Vd). It is these drugs which require a 'booster' loading dose.

MICRO-print

- For some drugs the loading dose can be given as a single dose, whereas others require the dose to be split.
- This can range from 2–3 doses over 24 hours (e.g. digoxin) to a longer titration regimen such as is seen with amiodarone.
- Splitting is required if administering a single large dose would lead to transiently toxic plasma levels before compartmental distribution occurs.

PRINCIPLES OF LOADING DOSES

- Administering loading doses is safe provided there is understanding of the basic principles.
- It must be noted that elimination has no bearing on loading doses, as illustrated by its absence from the following equation.

$$\text{Loading dose} = \text{desired therapeutic concentration} \times \text{Vd}$$

- Elimination (e.g. renal clearance) should therefore not be taken into account when determining the appropriate loading dose.

Clinical pharmacology

- The above equation also demonstrates that loading dose calculation is based upon a linear scale (i.e. double the dose, double the level). This principle is demonstrated by the Bucket Rule analogy.

MICRO-facts

The 'Bucket Rule'

Imagine a patient as a 5 litre bucket. To reach therapeutic levels the bucket must be filled with the drug (water). Now imagine the elimination of this drug (water) is via a hole in the bottom of the bucket.

Irrespective of the size of the hole, it still takes 5 litres to fill ('load') the bucket!

What changes is how much and how often you have to top it up with in order to keep it full, and that is the maintenance dose!

MICRO-case

The fictional drug 'Levojate' has a half-life of 50 hours, and a high Vd. It is hepatically metabolised and renally excreted. It is used for both acute and long-term management of severe cardiac arrhythmias. For these pharmacokinetic reasons it requires a loading dose of 10 mg/kg, and the therapeutic range is 1–2 mg/L.

Mr Smith is admitted to the Emergency Department (ED) with shortness of breath due to a severe arrhythmia, and requires Levojate, which he has never had before. He is 70 kg in weight, of a forgetful disposition and has chronic kidney disease.

$$\text{Loading dose} = 10 \times 70 = 700 \text{ mg}$$

Following administration of the dose he returns to sinus rhythm. Serum plasma levels return as 1.5 mg/L confirming appropriate dosing. He is put on an appropriate maintenance dose and is soon discharged from hospital.

Two weeks later he is admitted again with a severe arrhythmia. He admits that he has sometimes forgotten to take his tablets. The doctors do a random blood test and it shows a plasma level of 0.75 mg/L.

To determine the appropriate management consider the linearity of loading doses.

Reloading dose calculation:

Desired plasma concentration = 1. 5 mg/L (normal range 1–2 mg/L)

Actual plasma concentration = 0.75 mg/L

continued...

continued...

Current plasma concentration at steady state is half what it should be. To fill 'the Bucket' he needs a top up of half the loading dose.

Calculating loading dose = 10 mg/kg/2 = 5 mg/kg

Therefore appropriate loading dose: 5 × 70 = 350 mg

Key learning points

- Loading doses are a booster dose to get long acting drugs up to therapeutic range.
- Elimination is not a factor in loading doses.
- Loading doses are calculated on a linear scale whether the drugs are eliminated by first- or zero-order metabolism.
- Maintenance dosing requires consideration of elimination and steady-state concentrations (see Section 2.3).

2.3 MAINTENANCE DOSING

- Maintenance doses are the normal daily dose (i.e. the 'top up' dose in the 'Bucket' analogy).
- This is often the same as the loading dose but for those drugs with a long half-life the maintenance dose can be very much smaller.
- Unlike loading doses, calculating maintenance doses requires consideration of multiple factors:
    - Relationship of steady state and elimination
        - Once at steady state a drug will be fully distributed throughout the body as defined by its V_d.
        - At this point the plasma concentration is only affected by the balance between the rate of administration and the rate of elimination.
- Concentration at steady state (C_{ss}) = rate of administration/clearance.

MICRO-facts

For any change in administration or elimination when at steady state, (e.g. change of dose or renal function) it will take time for plasma levels to reach a constant due to redistribution of drug between the plasma and second (or third) compartment.

This time will again be 4–5 half-lives of the drug.

continued...

continued...

- Metabolism and elimination
  - From the above equation it can be seen that the concentration at steady state is proportional to the dose and elimination (first order kinetics).
  - In most cases this presumption is true, meaning a linear response is seen between the dose administered and the plasma concentration at steady state (i.e. 'double the maintenance dose, double the Css').
  - If however the metabolism or excretory pathways can be saturated, 'non-linear' zero order kinetics will apply at dosing above this level.
- Above this point a dose increase leads to an exponential rise in Css.

MICRO-facts

For calculation of maintenance doses:

- First order kinetics: Double the dose, double the level
- Zero order kinetics: Small incremental changes for prescribing maintenance doses

2.4 THERAPEUTIC DRUG MONITORING

For advice on loading doses for therapeutic drug monitoring see the loading dose section.

- Plasma drug level monitoring is usually required for drugs where there is:
  - A narrow therapeutic range, i.e. narrow range of therapeutic efficacy between 'no effect' and 'toxicity' (Ch. 1, Fig. 1.4).
  - A risk of accumulation leading to toxicity.
- Consideration of many of the above principles is necessary when calculating appropriate drug dosing.

Specific factors are discussed next.

DRUG PROPERTIES

- Both the pharmacodynamic and kinetic properties of a drug determine whether drug levels should be monitored.
- Pharmacodynamic effects depend upon the minimum effective concentration and maximum concentration before toxicity. This influences how closely you must monitor plasma levels to ensure no loss of efficacy or potential toxicity.
- Pharmacokinetics affect dosing frequency. If these are altered (for example with renally excreted drugs in renal failure) then allowance must be given for longer drug clearance or accumulation will lead to toxicity.

Clinical pharmacology

- These factors influence the timing of drug administration, as demonstrated in the MICRO-case below.

MICRO-case

The fictional drug 'Cipromull' has a half-life of 12 hours and is normally given at a dose of 50 mg BD. The therapeutic effect is seen at peak serum levels above 1 mg/L. Toxicity occurs with peak levels above 2 mg/L (peak serum therapeutic range 1–2 mg/L). Minimum levels must be maintained to ensure efficacy throughout the day. Examples of the drug's profile with varying patient weight and renal function can be seen in Figures 2.2 through 2.4.

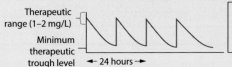

Therapeutic range (1–2 mg/L)

Minimum therapeutic trough level ← 24 hours →

Rx 50 mg BD
This dose ensures therapeutic efficacy throughout the day without periods of toxicity or sub-therapeutic levels.

Fig. 2.2 Ideal case: normal weight patient, normal renal function.

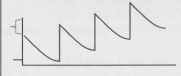

Rx 50 mg BD
Initial dose is insufficient due to large size, however due to the reduced renal function he accumulates drug and becomes toxic.

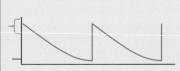

Solution - Rx 100 mg OD
A larger dose ensures efficacy with each dose. A reduced frequency of administration (here given daily) avoids accumulation.

Fig. 2.3 Body builder: heavy weight, poor renal function.

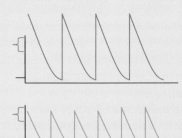

Rx 50 mg BD
Normal dose leads to toxicity, but is cleared by the kidneys.

Solution - Rx 25 mg TDS
Smaller dose avoids toxicity, and increased frequency of administration ensures efficacy throughout the day.

Fig. 2.4 Elderly lady: small frame, light weight, normal renal function.

TIMING OF DOSES AND PLASMA LEVELS

- Critically important, particularly with maintenance doses where you are trying to calculate an effective long-term dose, not just 'boost' levels as in loading.
- A plasma drug level is often meaningless without appropriate timing.
- Lab standards are set for each drug regarding timing of levels in relation to dose and these must be adhered to provide meaningful drug levels that can be used to alter drug dosing.
- Consideration must be paid to the relationship to steady state. If the levels taken do not represent steady-state concentrations, you cannot predict the response using the normal linear calculation.
- For example: if the level is taken prior to steady state a low level may be seen when in fact a few days later a plasma level may show therapeutic range (see Ch. 1, Fig. 1.3). In this case a dose increase would be inappropriate and may lead to toxicity.

Clinical pharmacology

3 Pharmacodynamics

Pharmacodynamics can be considered the aspect of pharmacology concerned with 'what the drug does to the body', i.e. how drugs elicit their actions and also adverse effects.

3.1 BASIC PRINCIPLES OF DRUG ACTION

- For the majority of drugs, the mechanisms of action can be broadly characterized into two categories.
  - Non-specific mechanisms
  - Specific mechanisms
    - Site-specific non-receptor mechanisms
    - Receptor mechanisms

NON-SPECIFIC MECHANISMS

- These drugs exhibit their action through a variety of mechanisms but do not interact with any of the body's receptors (discussed further below).
- The mechanisms are non-specific and due to simple chemical or physical interactions.
- Examples include:
  - Osmotic laxatives (e.g. lactulose) draw water into the gut thereby softening stools.
  - Bulk forming laxatives are not absorbed and simply 'bulk' up the contents of the intestines resulting in a softer stool.
  - Antacids directly neutralize stomach acid therefore reducing the pH.
- Cholestyramine binds bile acids (and some other drugs), reducing their absorption from the GI tract.

SPECIFIC MECHANISMS

- The majority of drugs exert their effect via mechanisms within this category.
- These drugs attach to specific macromolecular proteins to elicit their effect.
  - These proteins are of the following types:
    - Receptors (various subcategories described below)
    - Enzymes

     – Ion channels
     – Transport systems
- Many factors that influence drug–protein binding are the same regardless of the type of protein and are discussed further below.

Drug–protein binding
Specificity of binding

- The binding of a drug to protein is usually highly specific due to the steric (shape) nature of the complex.
- The shape of the chemical ligand (drug or endogenous mediator) is specific to the active site of the macromolecular protein (commonly referred to as the 'lock and key interaction').
- If the ligand binds only one type of protein it is 'specific'. If it preferentially binds one, but also affects others it is said to be 'selective'.
- Drug binding to other receptors than those targeted (i.e. non-specificity) is one mechanism by which adverse effects occur.

Drug–protein interactions

- Drug–protein binding is subject to numerous biochemical interactions.
- The nature of these interactions affects the pharmacodynamic and subsequent clinical effects of the drug.
  - Affinity: How tightly the ligand binds the protein.
  - Efficacy: Clinical response in relation to proportion of 'receptors' bound by a ligand.
  - Potency: Proportional to affinity and efficacy, i.e. a potent drug is one with high affinity and efficacy producing effects at low concentrations (Fig. 3.2).
- The type of chemical interaction is also important.
  - Irreversible covalent bonds between the drug and protein receptor are extremely strong and cannot be overcome.
- Weaker chemical interactions (i.e. van der Waals or hydrogen bonds) mean that the binding can be overcome if subject to other forces. This leads to reversible binding.

Mechanisms of clinical effects

- The clinical effects of drug–protein interactions are dependent upon the nature of the interaction.

Agonists

- When an agonistic drug binds to a receptor it will elicit a positive response (i.e. it will activate that receptor).

Variable effects of agonists

- Most agonists produce a positive response upon activation of a receptor.

- This positive response may be less, equal or more than the endogenous mediator.
  - Super agonists produce a greater maximal response. Clinical examples are rare.
  - Full agonists produce an equivalent maximal response.
  - Partial agonists (such as buprenorphine) never lead to a maximal effect even in the presence of high concentrations. This mechanism is explained below in the section 'Spare receptors'.
- Inverse agonists produce a response opposite to the endogenous mediator. Again these are rare in clinical practice.

Antagonists

- These drugs reduce the response to an endogenous mediator.
- This effect may be achieved in a number of ways:
  - Pharmacological antagonism: Blocking the endogenous mediator from binding with the receptor via either competitive or irreversible processes as explained above. This is the most common mechanism.
  - Physiological antagonism: Where the drug causes an opposing effect.
  - Chemical antagonism: The drug interacts with another ligand preventing it from binding with the receptor.

Irreversible and competitive antagonism

- Irreversible interactions cannot be overcome. For example, the inhibition of cyclooxygenase (COX) by aspirin.
  - Affected platelets have their COX irreversibly inhibited.
  - Platelets cannot produce further COX, therefore they are deactivated for the duration of their life.
  - On cessation of the aspirin, the anti-platelet effect will persist until new platelets have been produced despite there being no drug in the body.
- In comparison, reversible interactions may be overcome.
  - Weaker chemical interactions result in transient association and dissociation of the drug with the protein.
  - In this scenario, if two or more ligands compete for the same binding site, the one with the higher concentration has the greater probability of combining with the receptor to elicit its effect.
- Clinically this means that drugs and endogenous mediators compete for protein occupancy, and whoever has the highest concentration wins. This is known as 'competitive antagonism'.

Slow processes

- Persistent binding of some receptors after more prolonged exposure to a drug may alter the clinical response.

Clinical pharmacology

- This may occur relatively quickly due to desensitisation of the receptor (tachyphylaxis).
  - For example, regular use of nitrates requires a 'nitrate free period' to ensure continued effect of the drug.
  - Accordingly, nitrates are not normally prescribed in the evening.
- It may also occur more slowly, with increased (up-regulation), or decreased (down-regulation) receptor production.
  - Prolonged use of beta-blockers leads to up-regulation of receptor production. Consequently abrupt cessation of beta-blockers can cause rebound tachycardia as the increased number of receptors are bound by the now un-blocked endogenous mediator.
- Decongestants such as pseudoephedrine and xylometazoline cause vasoconstriction mediated by alpha-adrenoceptors. Prolonged use leads to down-regulation and rebound congestion.

Clinical response of drug–protein interactions

- For the majority of drugs the clinical effect is directly related to the plasma concentration which can be visualised using a concentration versus effect (Fig. 3.1).
- This demonstrates that the clinical effect is hyperbolic compared to the dose.
- As the dose increases the rate of change in clinical effect reduces until a plateau is reached. This usually represents progressive saturation of receptor sites.
  - Note the semi-logarithmic representation is commonly used, simply because it aids pharmacological analysis.
- Upon activation of a 'ligand-protein complex', the clinical response depends upon the pharmacodynamic nature of the drug (Fig. 3.2).
  - A potent drug may produce 100% effect at low concentrations (curve A).

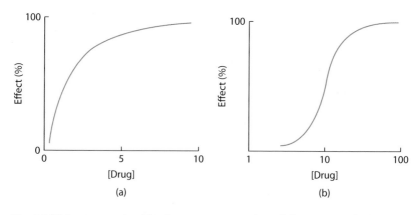

Fig. 3.1 The concentration (dose)-response curve plotted showing actual physiological response, and semi-logarithmic display.

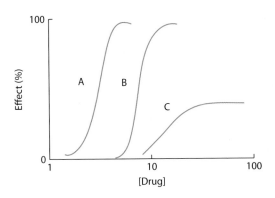

Fig. 3.2 Concentration (dose)-response curves representing drugs with potencies decreasing from A–C.

- Curve B represents a drug with high efficacy (can reach 100% effect), but a lower affinity. A higher concentration is therefore required, and drug B is said to be less potent than drug A.
- Curve C represents a drug with a low potency, low affinity (high concentration required for effect) and low efficacy (cannot achieve 100% effect). When acting on receptors, these drugs are also known as *partial agonists* as described below.

MICRO-print

Spare receptors

- Super agonists may cause 100% effect with a small amount of receptor occupancy, which leaves many 'spare receptors'.
- Partial agonists can never lead to 100% effect even at 100% receptor occupancy.
- This is of note when partial agonists and full agonists compete for receptor occupancy, i.e. a partial agonist may competitively reduce a full agonists effect.

Receptor mechanisms

- A receptor is a macromolecular protein in a cell which is the site of action for a specific endogenous mediator such as transmitter or hormone.
- Each receptor is linked to a mechanism that results in a cellular response. These different systems can be subdivided into four 'super families' of receptors (Fig. 3.3).

Ligand gated ion channels

- These receptors are linked to a transmembrane ion channel leading to a rapid response (milliseconds).

Clinical pharmacology

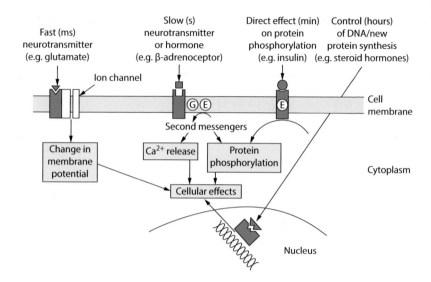

Fig. 3.3 Receptor types with associated cellular mechanisms.

- Many neurotransmitters use this system including GABA, serotonin and nicotinic ACh.
- Note this is different to voltage gated ion channels that are discussed further below.

G-protein coupled receptors

- These receptors are linked to a transmembrane G-protein.
- Activation of the extracellular receptor switches 'on' the G-protein, leading to a cascade of intracellular 'second messengers' which induce an intracellular effect. This is often mediated by associated enzymes.
- This process is slower than ion channels (seconds).
- Common second messengers include Ca^{2+} and cyclic adenosine monophosphate (cAMP).

Enzyme linked receptors

- These have an intrinsic intracellular enzyme with relatively slow response times.
- Examples include the insulin receptor.

Intranuclear receptors

- These receptors within the nucleus of the cell regulate transcription and protein synthesis.
- This process takes time and so the response is seen hours after receptor activation.

MICRO-print
Steroid receptors

- Steroid receptors are intranuclear.
- In the treatment of anaphylaxis, adrenaline is used for immediate effect associated with the IgE mediated type 1 hypersensitivity reaction.
- Corticosteroids such as prednisolone or hydrocortisone are used to ameliorate subsequent immune activity, and may reduce mast cell degranulation associated with the bisphasic nature of the immune response.

Site-specific non-receptor mechanisms

- Some drugs work at specific sites which are not classed as receptors as they are not sites for specific binding of endogenous mediators.
- These include enzymes and transport systems.

Enzyme interactions

- Enzymes are catalysts for chemical processes.
- Drugs may affect enzymatic function by specific interaction with the enzyme substrate site.
- This interaction is subject to the same principles of all specific mechanisms as discussed above.
- Almost all drug-enzyme interactions involve blocking of substrate binding and therefore reduction in enzymatic function. Common examples include:
  - Acetylcholinesterase inhibitors (for example, **neostigmine** for myasthenia gravis or **rivastigmine** for Alzheimer's disease).
  - Monoamine oxidase inhibitors (for example, **phenelzine** for depression).
  - Dihydrofolate reductase inhibitor (for example, **methotrexate** used for autoimmune diseases and oncological chemotherapy).

Transporters

- Transport systems enable molecules to cross hydrophobic cell membranes.
- Broadly speaking there are two types: ion channels (voltage gated) and active transport systems.

Ion channels (voltage gated)

- These proteins act as channels or pores that selectively allow charged ions to cross the cell membrane down the electrochemical gradient.
- Most drugs work by blocking these ion channels and therefore preventing electrochemical changes.

Clinical pharmacology

- Common ion channels involved include Na⁺, K⁺ and Ca²⁺.
  - Local anaesthetics such as lidocaine work by blocking Na⁺ entry into neurones preventing their electrical conduction.
  - Calcium (Ca²⁺) is required for smooth (e.g. vasculature) and cardiac muscle contraction and is also involved in AV conduction within the heart.
    - Calcium channel blockers may exhibit different effects depending on which type of calcium channel they selectively block.
- This can include reduction in peripheral vascular resistance, anti-anginal effect, reduce myocardial work (negative ionotrope) or slow AV conduction (negative chronotrope).

MICRO-print

Types of ion channels

- Ion channels while similar in structure differ in their activation.
- Some are simply pores allowing charged ions to pass through the hydrophobic membrane (*voltage gated ion channels*).
- For others ion transfer is controlled by ligand (or drug) binding to the channels extra-cellular domain. These are known as *ligand gated ion channels*. As these 'gates' are sites for endogenous mediators these are classified as true receptor sites.
- Some channels may incorporate both voltage and ligand gated elements.

Active transport systems

- These processes require energy provided by the ubiquitous ATPase (adenosine triphosphatase).
- This energy is used to drive ions and molecules across cell membranes, against their concentration gradient.
- The transport systems require a pump which creates a gradient. There are broadly two mechanisms involved here:
  - Direct: Seen in 'active transport' systems such as the H⁺/K⁺ATPase pump (or Proton pump) upon which PPI's act (see Ch. 7, Section 7.1).
  - Indirect: Co-transport where the pump provides a gradient for movement of other molecules. An example being furosemide (see Ch. 5, Section 5.2) which works on the NKCC2 co-transport channel moving Na⁺, K⁺ and Cl⁻ ions across a cell membrane, the electrochemical gradient for this being provided by the Na⁺/K⁺ATPase pump.

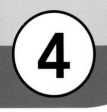

4 Drug handling by the body

4.1 DRUG ROUTE AND ABSORPTION

There are several routes of administration, each of which may be used for specific purposes. Each route will have its own advantages and disadvantages. The main routes are discussed below.

ORAL ROUTE

- Lipophilic non-ionized drugs are more readily absorbed through the GI tract (mostly the small intestine).
- The percentage of drug reaching the systemic circulation (bioavailability) is dependent on multiple factors (see Fig. 4.1):
    - The degree of lipid solubility (lipophilicity) of the drug.
    - Drug inactivation or binding throughout the GI tract.
    - 'First-pass metabolism' (inactivation by the liver after passage through the portal vein).
- Some drugs may be given orally for a local effect on the gastrointestinal tract with negligible systemic absorption. For example:
    - **Budesonide** and 5-ASA for the treatment of IBD.
    - **Vancomycin** for *Clostridium difficile*.
    - **Lactulose** for constipation.

> ## MICRO-facts
>
> ### Artificial alteration of absorption
> - Modified release (MR) (sometimes known as slow release [SR] or controlled release [CR]) preparations usually contain drug in a matrix form which slowly releases the drug along its passage through the GI tract.
> - This may reduce peak concentrations and artificially extend the action of drugs with a short half-life.
> - However, absorption of the drug is often incomplete, reducing the apparent bioavailability.
> - This can be particularly important when changing drug forms in very dose-sensitive conditions such as Parkinson's disease.
>
> *continued…*

continued...

- Dose alterations must be considered when switching, for example modified release preparations of levodopa compounds have a 30–50% reduction in bioavailability compared to the standard release formulations.
- Enteric Coated (EC) preparations are usually pH sensitive weakly acidic coatings which resist breakdown within the stomach, protecting the drug from degradation.
- In the alkaline pH of the small intestine, however, they dissolve and release the drug for absorption.

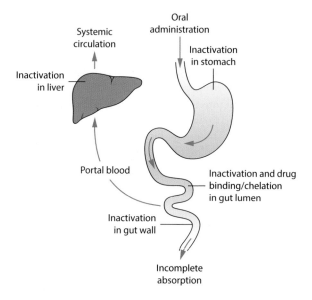

Fig. 4.1 Factors affecting bioavailability after oral administration.

PARENTERAL ROUTES

These routes bypass any absorption barriers for the drug which results in a bioavailability of 100%.

Intravenous

- Drug enters directly into the circulation allowing:
  - Rapid effect.
  - Continuous infusion (for titrating doses or drugs with very short half-lives).
- Efficacy if the oral route is not suitable (for example if the drug is not absorbed or the patient is nil by mouth).

Intramuscular and subcutaneous

- These routes allow easy administration of single doses of drugs.
- Absorption into systemic circulation is affected by blood flow, which is dependent upon peripheral perfusion.
- Cutaneous blood flow is lower than muscular hence slower absorption.
- This delayed absorption may provide a sustained effect, but can also delay the onset of action.
- Subcutaneous injection:
  - Usually well tolerated.
  - However, with longer term injection to the same site lipodystrophy may occur, particularly with insulin.
- Intramuscular injection:
  - Often helpful in the absence of IV access.
  - However, it can be painful, particularly with volumes greater than 1–2 mL.
  - Haematoma is a potential complication and may lead to abscess formation.
  - Consequently, this route should be avoided in those with coagulopathy or concurrent anticoagulation.

BUCCAL, SUBLINGUAL AND RECTAL

- These routes are often useful for patients for whom oral administration is not appropriate.
- Examples include:
  - A patient suffering from a seizure who is unconscious with no IV access may be administered buccal **midazolam**.
  - **Diclofenac** suppositories for those undergoing anaesthesia.
- The main advantages of these techniques are that they avoid 'first-pass' metabolism, and are frequently used for drugs which administered orally would have low bioavailability. Common examples are **glycerol trinitrate** and **fentanyl**.
- Onset of action is also more rapid compared to oral.

TOPICAL

- This route may be used for local action such as with creams and ointments.
- Patches are increasingly used for systemic dosing as an alternative to oral administration.
- The main considerations are:
  - Bypassing of first-pass metabolism.
  - Potential for local side effects, most commonly itching.
  - Variable absorption dependant on skin hydration and temperature.
- Common systemic examples are **glyceryl trinitrate, fentanyl** and **nicotine**.

Clinical pharmacology

4.2 METABOLISM

Drug metabolism within the body varies dependent on the drug, the route of administration and an individual's physiology.

DRUG FACTORS

- The nature of the metabolism depends upon the chemical properties of a drug.
- Most drugs are excreted by the kidneys, which require them to be water soluble (ionized) to allow diffusion across the tubular membrane.
- Drugs which are water soluble such as lisinopril may therefore be excreted unchanged in the urine, whereas others require extensive metabolism.

Metabolism as a function

- The function of metabolism is to allow elimination, and the resultant metabolites are frequently less active than the parent drug.
- This process, however, may also yield other effects if the metabolites are themselves active.
- Metabolism does not necessarily mean inactivation. This is explained in the examples below.
- Prodrugs:
  - These drugs require metabolism from the administered form into the active compound.
  - This process may be used for therapeutic effect, for example:
    - **Levodopa** is an inactive precursor converted to the active dopamine by dopa-decarboxylase.
    - Both of these compounds cross the blood brain barrier delivering active dopamine to the brain after metabolism.
    - To prevent systemic conversion leading to side effects without central benefit, levodopa is co-administered with a dopa-decarboxylase inhibitor which does not cross the blood brain barrier.
    - In this way the prodrug has been used to selectively target the organ in which its action is required for PD patients.
- Active metabolites:
  - The action of atorvastatin is extended by the production of these compounds.
  - **Atorvastatin** may therefore be given at any time of the day, whereas **simvastatin** must be administered at night when most HMG co-reductase A is most active and most cholesterol is produced.
- Toxic metabolites:
  - In **paracetamol** overdose the major metabolism pathways become saturated leading to increased production of a toxic intermediate of a minor pathway called NAPQI, which is detoxified by glutathione conjugation.

- Once glutathione supply is depleted, toxic NAPQI builds up resulting in toxicity including hepatocellular necrosis.

ROUTE FACTORS

- As previously discussed, oral administration may result in significant 'first-pass' metabolism and a failure to achieve systemically therapeutic levels.
- Other routes of administration bypassing this process must be sought.

PHYSIOLOGICAL FACTORS

- The liver is the principal organ of drug metabolism and here drugs may undergo two separate episodes of metabolism (Phase I and Phase II).
- Metabolism may be affected by liver function and genetic make-up.
- Liver function is difficult to ascertain as it is dependent upon blood flow, hepatocyte function and metabolizing enzyme capacity.
- There is no test (including LFTs) available that will accurately assess liver function. In liver failure PT is a reasonable proxy for the liver's synthetic function.
- Individuals may have differing levels of the metabolic CYP450 enzymes (discussed below), altering their metabolism potential. Low function *poor metabolizers* will be prone to drug toxicity.

Hepatic metabolism
Phase I metabolism

- This process chemically alters the drugs by oxidation, hydrolysis or reduction, and produces the inactive or active metabolites.
- This is mediated within the endoplasmic reticulum of the hepatocytes by a number of related enzymes known as cytochrome P450 (CYP450).
- Following this phase, the metabolites may then be excreted or undergo further Phase II metabolism.
- Interactions between drugs may occur if they compete for metabolism with the same enzyme group, potentially leading to toxicity due to reduced metabolism.
- Some drugs increase (induce) or decrease (inhibit) the function of these enzymes which can lead to alterations in drug metabolism (see below).

Phase II metabolism

- This process conjugates the drug or phase I metabolite with a water soluble compound such as glucuronic acid, acetate, amino acids or methionine.
- This enhances water solubility to aid excretion and invariably also inactivates the compound.

Enzyme induction and inhibition

- If a drug induces a certain CYP450 enzyme it will increase its function therefore enhancing metabolism of any drug substrate.

- In this way it will tend to decrease the effect of that drug.
- Conversely enzyme inhibition will tend to increase the function of the effected drug by reducing metabolism.
  - Carbamazepine is an auto-inducer. It enhances the activity of CYP3A4, an enzyme which metabolizes itself. It therefore enhances its own metabolism.
- Common drugs affected by enzyme inhibition and induction are:
  - **Theophylline/aminophylline**
  - **Warfarin**
  - **Phenytoin**
  - **Carbamazepine**

Table 4.1 **Enzyme inducers and inhibitors**

INDUCERS	INHIBITORS
Rifampicin	Sodium valproate
Ethanol (chronic)	Isoniazid
Spironolactone	Cimetidine
Phenytoin	Ketoconazole
Barbiturates	Fluconazole
Carbamazepine	Amiodarone and Atorvastatin
Griseofulvin	Chloramphenicol
	Erythromycin/macrolides
	Sulphonylureas (e.g. gliclazide)
	Ciprofloxacin
	Omeprazole
	Metronidazole

MICRO-facts

Mnemonics for enzyme inducers and inhibitors

Mnemonics can be created to aid memory of the common drugs involved:

- R_E_S_P_'B'_C_'G' – find out what 'induces' me
  - Think turberculosis, respiratory problems and BCG vaccine, to Aretha Franklin.
- SICKFACES.COM 'inhibits' my will to drink!
- Acute alcohol also enzyme inhibitor.

> **MICRO-print**
> **Alcohol and effects on hepatic metabolism**
> - Alcohol is predominately metabolized in the liver by alcohol dehydrogenase, and to a lesser extent by CYP2E1.
> - CYP2E1 is induced in chronic alcohol intake leading to increased tolerance, and subsequently increasing metabolism of other drugs metabolized by this enzyme.
> - Acute alcohol intake, however, competitively inhibits metabolism of drugs metabolized by similar pathways.

4.3 EXCRETION

The most important organ of excretion is the kidney; however some drugs are excreted in the bile. Pulmonary excretion is the route for elimination of volatile anaesthetics.

RENAL EXCRETION

- Most drugs are renally excreted, requiring them to be water soluble, as lipid soluble drugs are freely reabsorbed through the renal tubules removing them from the urine.
- Lipid soluble drugs must therefore undergo metabolism as outlined above to be removed.

> **MICRO-print**
> **pH associated renal excretion**
> - pH associated dissociation of acids and bases denotes that a weak acid will exist in its unionized form in acidic solution, and the converse is true for bases.
> - These unionized forms are more readily reabsorbed through the renal tubules, out of the urine.
> - Altering the urine's pH may therefore increase excretion.
> - In the overdose of the weakly acidic aspirin, sodium bicarbonate may be used to alkalinize the urine and therefore increase excretion.

BILIARY EXCRETION

- This is the only other significant form of excretion besides renal.
- Drugs with a high molecular weight, particularly those conjugated with glucuronic acid are more likely to be excreted in this way.

Clinical pharmacology

- These conjugated molecules may be cleaved in the intestines by the floral bacteria, allowing the drug to be reabsorbed. This is known as the entero-hepatic circulation.
- With reduced bacteria levels less reabsorption would take place, decreasing drug levels in the body.
- Via this mechanism many oestrogen based oral contraceptive pills are rendered ineffective when used in combination with antibiotics.

MICRO-reference
The MERCK Manuals. Drug excretion. Whitehouse Station, NJ, USA. 2013. Available from: http://www.merckmanuals.com/professional/clinical_pharmacology/pharmacokinetics/drug_excretion.html

---

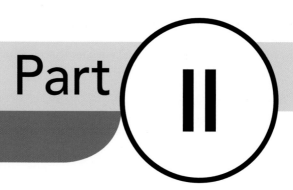

Part II

Drugs and practical prescribing

5 Cardiovascular drugs

5.1 POSITIVE INOTROPES

CARDIAC GLYCOSIDES (DIGOXIN)

Pharmacodynamics

- Inhibits Na^+/K^+ ATPase in cardiac and other tissues.
- Subsequent increased intracellular Na^+ affects the Na^+/Ca^{2+} transporter leading to a net increase in intracellular Ca^{2+}.
- Higher calcium levels at the time of excitation produce a positive inotropic effect (increased myocardial contractility).
- Autonomic nervous system actions results in increased vagal tone and reduced conduction through atria and AV node reducing the ventricular rate.

> **MICRO-facts**
>
> K^+ and digoxin compete for binding at the Na^+/K^+ ATPase therefore hypokalaemia increases effects of digoxin.

Pharmacokinetics

- Absorption:
    - 70% oral bioavailability (tablet).
    - IV effects seen within 5–30 minutes, peak effect at 1–5 hours.
    - Oral preparation has initial effect within 2 hours, peak effect within 6 hours.
    - 125 micrograms tablet = 100 micrograms syrup = 100 micrograms IV preparation.
- Elimination:
    - Renal elimination of mostly unchanged drug.
    - $t_{1/2}$ 30–40 hours.

Indications

- Heart failure (± atrial fibrillation).
- Atrial fibrillation/atrial flutter.

Contraindications

- AV block (intermittent complete and second degree).
- Supraventricular tachycardia with an accessory pathway (e.g. Wolf-Parkinson syndrome).

> ## MICRO-facts
>
> Digoxin may enhance conduction through accessory pathways in conditions such as Wolf-Parkinson syndrome due to an increased refractory period in the AV node.

- Hypertrophic obstructive cardiomyopathy, ventricular tachycardia.
- Myocarditis, pericarditis.

Cautions

- Recent MI, sick sinus syndrome, thyroid disease, elderly patients, electrolyte disturbances, renal failure (reduce maintenance dose).

Adverse effects

- Cardiac conduction disturbance/arrhythmias: Almost any rhythm disturbance, including bigeminy/trigeminy, bradycardia, SVT (especially with AV block), high grade AV block or ventricular tachycardia.
- Visual disturbance: Yellow visual tinge (mild toxicity) and blurred vision.
- Gastrointestinal: Nausea/vomiting (sign of toxicity), diarrhoea, intestinal necrosis.
- Others: Gynaecomastia, depression, confusion, psychosis.

> MICRO-monitoring
> **Digoxin monitoring and toxicity**
> - Therapeutic drug monitoring: see Ch. 2, Section 2.4
>   - Therapeutic range: 0.8–2.0 mg/L.
>   - Levels timing: 6–8 hours post dose.
>   - Follows first order kinetics.
> - Approximately 7–10 days to steady state.

> ## MICRO-facts
>
> **Digoxin toxicity**
>
> - Toxicity is likely above 2 micrograms/L and almost inevitable over 3 micrograms/L.
>
> *continued...*

continued...

- Toxic symptoms may present even at normal serum concentrations in the presence of hypokalaemia (see above).
- Signs and symptoms:
  - Palpitations (may cause almost any arrhythmia).
  - Nausea/anorexia, diarrhoea.
  - Confusion.
  - Visual disturbance – blurred vision, yellow tinge.
- **DigiFab®** is a treatment using digoxin-specific antibody fragments which may be administered if there is haemodynamic instability associated with either:
  - Ventricular arrhythmias.
  - Bradyarrhythmias unresponsive to atropine.

Important interactions

- Pharmacokinetic:
  - Increased plasma concentrations: **Amiodarone, propafenone, quinidine, spironolactone**, macrolide/tetracycline antibiotics, **gentamicin, verapamil**.
- Pharmacodynamic:
  - Reduced cardiac conduction: Class I/III antiarrhythmics, non-dihydropyridine calcium channel blockers.
  - Predisposition to hypokalaemia: Loop/thiazide diuretics.

Examples

- Loading dose:
  - Normally 750–1500 micrograms (0.75–1.5) mg over 24 hours (including renal impairment).
  - Total 24-hour dose 15 mg/kg of ideal body weight, in 2–3 divided doses.
- Maintenance dose:
  - Normally 125–250 micrograms OD, oral.
  - Approximate maintenance dose requirements will be one-third of loading dose (reduced in renal impairment).

MICRO-reference
electronic Medicines Compendium (eMC). Digoxin Tablets BP 125 micrograms. Summary of product characteristics. Available from: http://www.medicines.org.uk/emc/medicine/23943/SPC/

Drugs and practical prescribing

5.2 DIURETICS

THIAZIDE DIURETICS

Pharmacodynamics

- Inhibit reabsorption of sodium and chloride ions in the distal convoluted tubules (DCT) of the kidney by blocking the Na^+Cl^- symporter therefore promoting diuresis.
- Also produces low serum potassium.
- High serum uric acid concentrations (hyperuricaemia) may occur due to competitive renal tubular secretion.
- Increased reabsorption of calcium leads to high serum levels.
- Anti-hypertensive effect not fully understood, may have an effect on renal prostaglandin synthesis as with loop diuretics.

Indications

- Hypertension.
- Oedema.
  - Used synergistically with loop diuretics.
    - The combined reduction in reabsorption at the loop of Henle and DCT produces profound diuresis.
- Prevention of renal calculi: Increased reabsorption of calcium reduces hypercalciuria.

Contraindications

- Persistent hypokalaemia/hyponatraemia.
- Symptomatic hyperuricaemia.
- Addison's disease.
- Hypercalcaemia.

Cautions

- Renal impairment and nephrotic syndrome.
- May exacerbate diabetes, gout and SLE.
- Electrolyte disturbances (see above).
- Also malnutrition, hyperaldosteronism and hepatic impairment.

Adverse effects

- Postural hypotension: May be significant, especially in elderly patients.
- Electrolyte disturbance: Hypokalaemia, hyponatraemia, hypomagnesaemia, hypercalcaemia and hypochloraemic alkalosis.
- Hyperuricaemia/gout: See Pharmacodynamics, above.
- Others: Pancreatitis, cholestasis, headache, visual disturbance, hypersensitivity, dyslipidaemias, paraesthesia, blood disorders.

Important interactions
- Increases plasma concentrations of lithium.
- NSAIDs reduce diuretic effect by inhibiting prostaglandin synthesis.
- Risk of first dose hypotension with ACEis/ARBs.
- Induced hypokalaemia potentiates digoxin and other antiarrhythmic toxicity.
- Enhanced hypotensive effect when used with other antihypertensives.

Examples
- **Bendroflumethiazide:** 2.5 mg OD, oral
- **Indapamide:** 2.5 mg OD, oral (M/R preparation also available, 1.5 mg, oral, OD)
- **Metolazone:** Thiazide-like diuretic used synergistically with loop diuretics
- Others: **Hydrochlorothiazide** (common in United States and Europe), **Chlortalidone, Cyclopenthiazide, Xipamide**

LOOP DIURETICS

Pharmacodynamics
- Inhibit the $Na^+/K^+/2Cl^-$ transporter in the luminal membrane of the thick ascending limb of the loop of Henle, preventing reabsorption of sodium and chloride ions.
- This leads to reduced water reabsorption and thus diuresis.
- Also reduces the positive electrostatic potential of the tubular lumen, and so decreases reabsorption of cations such as potassium, calcium and magnesium.
- Increases renal synthesis of prostaglandins, increasing renal blood flow and causing early venodilatation (this mechanism is inhibited by NSAIDs).
- Net effect is reduction in circulating volume and reduced venous preload.

Pharmacokinetics
- Absorption: Rapid absorption from gut; oral bioavailability of furosemide is variable around 65%. Bumetanide's is over 80% and more predictable (possibly more effective in presence of intestinal oedema).

Indications
- Oedema, including acute pulmonary oedema (may be used in combination with thiazides).
- Resistant hypertension.

Cautions and contraindications
- Electrolyte disturbances: (see below).
- Hypovolaemia, dehydration, anuria.
- Coma in hepatic failure.
- Renal failure secondary to nephrotoxic drugs.

Adverse effects

- Electrolyte disturbance: Hypokalaemia, (hypokalaemic metabolic alkalosis if severe). Hypomagnesaemia, hyponatraemia, hypocalcaemia and hypochloraemia also occur.
- Ototoxicity: Dose related, usually reversible.
- Hyperuricaemia/gout: Mechanism as per thiazides.
- Others: Postural hypotension, pancreatitis, hypersensitivity, interstitial nephritis, hepatic encephalopathy, visual disturbance, blood disorders and gynaecomastia (bumetanide).

Important interactions

- Increases plasma concentrations of lithium.
- NSAIDs reduce diuretic effect by inhibiting prostaglandin synthesis and may also induce AKI in volume-depleted patients.
- Risk of first dose hypotension with ACEis/ARBs increased with furosemide.
- Induced hypokalaemia potentiates digoxin and other antiarrhythmic toxicity.
- Increased risk of nephrotoxicity when administered with aminoglycosides or amphotericin.

Examples

- **Furosemide:** 40 mg OD, oral (20–120 mg daily used frequently).
    - IV preparation available. Doses greater than 80 mg should not exceed 4 mg/min.
- **Bumetanide:** 1–5 mg OD, oral.
- **Torasemide: Torem®.**

MICRO-print
Bumetanide is roughly 40 times more potent than furosemide.

- 1 mg bumetanide oral = 40 mg furosemide oral.

Special requirements

- In severe oedema, bowel oedema may reduce oral absorption and IV administration may be warranted.

POTASSIUM-SPARING DIURETICS

- These drugs provide a diuretic effect without promoting urinary excretion of potassium.
- The two classes, potassium sparing diuretics and aldosterone antagonists, have different mechanisms and uses as outlined below.

Pharmacodynamics

- Aldosterone antagonists:
    - Competitively antagonize the effects of aldosterone by binding to steroid receptor in the distal convoluted tubule.
    - This decreases sodium and water reabsorption and reduces potassium excretion.
    - Spironolactone also has marked anti-androgen properties resulting in adverse effects (eplerenone less so).
- Potassium-sparing diuretics:
    - Provide a weak diuretic effect through reduction in sodium reabsorption in distal tubule by direct antagonism of luminal Na^+ (ENaC) channels.
    - K^+ excretion is reduced as secretion is coupled with Na^+ transport.

Indications

- Aldosterone antagonists:
    - Congestive heart failure/left ventricular dysfunction.
    - Nephrotic syndrome.
    - Ascites.
    - Primary hyperaldosteronism.
- Potassium-sparing diuretics:
    - Oedema.
    - Potassium conservation (in combination with loop or thiazide diuretics).

Cautions and contraindications

- Hyperkalaemia.
- Renal dysfunction/anuria.
- Hyponatraemia/Addison's disease.

Adverse effects

- Electrolyte disturbance: Hyponatraemia and hyperkalaemia.
- GI disturbances: Abdominal pain, constipation, diarrhoea.
- Endocrine disturbance:
    - Seen with aldosterone antagonists (spironolactone more than eplerenone).
    - Including gynaecomastia, impotence, menstrual irregularities.

Important interactions

- Risk of hyperkalaemia with ACE inhibitors/ARBs and K^+ supplements.
- NSAIDs may reduce diuretic effects.

Examples

Aldosterone antagonists

- **Spironolactone (Aldactone®):** Heart failure 25–50 mg OD, other indications 100–200 mg.
    - Compound preparations with loops/thiazides available.
- **Eplerenone Inspra®:** 25–50 mg OD, oral.

Potassium sparing diuretics

- **Amiloride:** With other diuretics 5–10 mg OD, oral.
  - Compound preparations: **Co-amilofruse (furosemide), co-amilozide (hydrochlorothiazide), Navispare® (cyclopenthiazide).**
- **Triamterene (Dytac®):** Also available in compound preparations.

Special requirements

- Monitor serum potassium and creatinine concentration regularly.

OTHER DIURETICS

- **Mannitol:** Osmotic diuretic used to treat cerebral oedema and raised intra-ocular pressure.
- **Acetazolamide:** A carbonic anhydrase inhibitor. It is a weak diuretic, also used for mountain sickness prophylaxis and in eye drops for glaucoma.

5.3 ANTIARRHYTHMIC DRUGS

CLASSIFICATION OF DRUGS FOR ARRHYTHMIAS

- The treatment of arrhythmias depends heavily upon accurate electrocardiogram interpretation and correct diagnosis. This may well require expert assistance.
- Classification of drugs may be subdivided into two categories:
  1. Clinical Classification of drug actions. This is generally considered the more useful system.
     - Supraventricular (narrow complex): **Adenosine, verapamil, digoxin.**
     - Both supra and ventricular: **Amiodarone**, beta-blockers, **disopyramide, flecainide,** and **propafenone**.
     - Ventricular (broad complex): **Lidocaine.**
  2. Vaughan Williams Classification of drug actions. Classification based upon electrical effects on cardiac myocytes.
     - Class I: membrane-stabilization Na^+ channel antagonist.
       - (Ia) **procainamide, disopyramide,** (Ib) **lidocaine,** (Ic) **flecainide**.
     - Class II: Beta adrenoceptor antagonist:
       - **Atenolol, metoprolol, esmolol, bisprolol**
     - Class III: K^+ channel antagonist:
       - **Amiodarone** (also class I and II activity), **sotalol** (also class II activity);
     - Class IV: Calcium channel antagonist, e.g. **verapamil, diltiazem** (not dihydropyridines).
     - Class V: other mechanisms, e.g. **digoxin, adenosine, magnesium sulphate.**

TREATMENT ALGORITHM FOR ARRHYTHMIAS

- Treatment choice should be based upon interpretation of ECG findings.
- Associated tachycardias and haemodynamic stability affect treatment options.
- If the patient is unstable with any arrhythmia then the treatment is DC cardioversion.

Supraventricular (narrow complex) arrhythmias
Regular rhythm

- Vagal manoeuvers: First line is Valsalva and/or carotid sinus massage.
- **Adenosine:** Second line should terminate most paroxysmal SVTs.
  - Atrial flutter requires rate control, and will not be terminated by adenosine but underlying flutter waves will become evident.
  - However if the SVT classification is unknown, adenosine may slow the rate and expose atrial activity on ECG revealing diagnosis.
- **Verapamil:** Third line if adenosine contraindicated/above treatment fails.

Irregular rhythm

- Likely AF: Use beta blocker or diltiazem. Consider **digoxin/amiodarone** if heart failure.
- **Flecainide** may be used in prophylaxis of disabling paroxysmal AF.

Ventricular (broad complex) arrhythmias
Regular rhythm

- Ventricular tachycardia: **Amiodarone**.
- Exception is a supraventricular arrhythmia with bundle branch block which can appear similarly. If bundle branch block has been previously documented on ECG then treat as regular narrow complex arrhythmia.

Irregular rhythm

- Expert help required.
- Likely AF with bundle branch block, but may be AF with ventricular pre-excitation (e.g. in WPW syndrome) or torsade de pointes (treat with IV magnesium).

MICRO-reference
Pitcher D, Perkins G. Peri-arrest arrhythmias. *Resuscitation Guidelines 2010*. Resuscitation Council UK. Available from: http://www.resus.org.uk/pages/periarst.pdf

CLASSES OF ANTIARRHYTHMIC DRUGS

- Beta-blockers, calcium channel blockers and digoxin are discussed under their own drug classes.

Class I antiarrhythmics

- See above for classifications and uses.
- All should be used under expert supervision only, and are themselves potentially arrhythmogenic.
  - **Disopyramide:**
    - Used in the prevention/treatment of ventricular and supraventricular arrhythmias.
    - May exacerbate heart failure due to negative inotropic effects and causes hypotension.
    - Causes significant anticholinergic side effects and nausea.
  - **Lidocaine:**
    - Used IV in the treatment of ventricular arrhythmias, especially after MI.
  - **Flecainide:**
    - Mainly used for prophylaxis of severe symptomatic paroxysmal AF.
    - May be used PO/IV in ventricular tachyarrythmias resistant to treatment.
    - Negative inotropic effects limit use and contraindicate in heart failure.
- Contraindicated in haemodynamically significant valvular disease and atrial conduction defects.
  - **Propafenone** is similar.

> **MICRO-reference**
> Craig M, Pratt MD, et al. Cardiac Arrhythmia Suppression Trial (CAST).
> *Circulation.* 1995; 91: 245–247.

Adenosine

- Indications:
  - Cardioversion of supraventricular tachycardias.
  - Aid to diagnosis of narrow and broad complex tachycardias (e.g. atrial flutter).
  - Induction of a 'stress' state for myocardial perfusion imaging.
- Given as rapid bolus to inhibit atrioventricular nodal conduction.
- Given as 6 mg IV, with up to two further 12-mg boluses if no effect.

- Contraindicated in second/third degree heart block, sick sinus syndrome, long QT, severe decompensated heart failure, severe hypotension and COPD/asthma (bronchospasm).

MICRO-facts

Administration of adenosine

- If using adenosine forewarn the patients that they may feel a 'sense of impending doom' upon administration.
- It is important to inform them that this will be short lived due to the drugs very short half-life (less than 10 seconds).
- Ensure continuous ECG monitoring is present, and print off the rhythm strips as they are useful for later analysis of adenosine's effects (if any).

Amiodarone and related drugs

- Extremely effective antiarrhythmic used in both acute and chronic situations.
- Use is limited by severity of adverse effects (see below).

Pharmacodynamics

- Has multiple cardiac effects:
  - Main antiarrhythmic effect achieved by prolongation of the QT interval (class III antiarrhythmic effect) due to potassium channel blockade.
  - Blocks sodium channels (class I activity) and weakly blocks calcium channels (class IV activity).
  - Has weak anti-adrenergic activity.
- Broad spectrum of action leads to reduced heart rate and AV nodal conduction.

Pharmacokinetics

- Distribution/elimination.
  - Very high Vd due to tissue accumulation.
  - This results in a very long $t_{1/2}$ (around 50 days) with clinical effect maintained for 1–3 months after loading.

Indications

- Supraventricular and ventricular dysrhythmias (note in the acute setting IV may act relatively quickly).

Cautions and contraindications
- Cardiac: Bradycardia, heart block.
- Hepatic: See adverse effects.
- Thyroid disease: See adverse effects.
- Respiratory: See adverse effects; chest x-ray required before initiating therapy.

Adverse effects
- Thyroid dysfunction:
  - High iodine content and similar structure to T4, may result in hyperthyroidism.
  - Interferes with peripheral conversion of T4 to T3 which may result in hypothyroidism.
- Hepatic impairment: Hepatic transaminases are commonly transiently elevated, but hepatitis may also occur.
- Pulmonary fibrosis: Dose-related pulmonary toxicity (fibrosis, pneumonitis, bronchiolitis obliterans) usually occurring in patients on long term therapy.
- Photosensitivity: Photodermatitis including grey skin discolouration in sun exposed areas. Patients should be advised to take precautions against sun damage.
- Corneal deposits: Common but usually asymptomatic. Resolve on discontinuation.

Important interactions
- Numerous interactions, please refer to a reference text for a full list.
- Notably and commonly:
  - Risk of ventricular arrhythmias
    - Antidepressants (TCAs and some SSRIs).
    - Antipsychotics (1st generation, and some 2nd generation: QT prolongation).
    - Antibiotics (quinolones and macrolides).
  - AV block, bradycardia and myocardial depression: verapamil and beta-blockers.
  - Increased plasma concentrations of: Digoxin (halve digoxin dose), flecainide (halve flecanide dose), anticoagulants (increased warfarin and dabigatran concentration) and phenytoin (increased plasma concentration).
- Risk of myopathy increased with CYP3A4 metabolized statins (e.g. simvastatin).

Examples
- **Amiodarone (Cordarone X®):**
  - Loading doses required due to extensive distribution (both IV and oral).

- PO: 200 mg TDS 7/7, 200 mg BD 7/7 then 200 mg daily.
  - ○ Dose may be adjusted by specialist. Use lowest possible maintenance dose to control arrhythmia.
- IV: 5 mg/kg over >30 min (300 mg in emergency resuscitation).
  - ○ Requires ECG monitoring.
- **Dronedarone (Multaq®):** Related drug without iodine moieties.

Special requirements

- Measurement of U+Es, LFTs and TFTs required before initiation of treatment and at 6 monthly intervals.
- New or progressive cough or dyspnoea should lead to investigation of possible pneumonitis.
- Central venous route of administration preferred if infusion required as can cause pain/inflammation if infused peripherally. Follow bolus with a large volume flush.

5.4 ADRENOCEPTOR ANTAGONISTS

α-ADRENOCEPTOR BLOCKING DRUGS

There are several α-adrenoceptors which have mixed and overlapping effects.
- α_1-adrenoceptors: Several subcategories which are distributed in varying amounts throughout the body.
- Generally, agonism leads to smooth muscle contraction (in contrast to the β-adrenoceptors).
- This is of pharmacological relevance with regard to vasoconstriction and bladder sphincter constriction.
- α_2-adrenoceptors: Targeted by drugs such as clonidine.

Pharmacodynamics

- Alpha-blockers selectively antagonize adrenergic effects at smooth-muscle α_1-adrenoceptors leading to reduced muscle tone resulting in multiple effects including:
  - Vasodilation and reduced systemic vascular resistance.
  - Reduced prostatic tone and reduction in urinary outflow resistance.
- **Tamsulosin** and **Alfuzosin** have preferential selectivity for prostatic α_{1A} receptors and therefore may cause less hypotension.

Indications

- Cardiac: Hypertension (not tamsulosin).
- Urological: Benign prostatic hypertrophy (BPH).
- Others: Raynaud's phenomenon, phaeochromocytoma (phenoxybenzamine only).

Cautions and contraindications

- Postural hypotension (especially first dose).

Adverse effects

- Hypotension/postural hypotension: First dose should be taken prior to bed.
- Others: Meiosis, nasal congestion, impaired ejaculation, dry mouth, blurred vision, headache, tachycardia, hypersensitivity.

Examples and dosing

- **Doxazosin (Cardura®)** (MR preparation - **XL**): 1–16 mg OD, oral
- **Indoramin (Doralese®)**
- **Prazosin (Hypovase®)**
- **Terazosin (Hytrin®)**
- **Alfuzosin (Xatral®):** BPH only
- **Tamsulosin (Flomaxtra® XL):** BPH only. With **dutasteride (Combodart®)**.

MICRO-facts

Phaeochromocytoma

Phenoxybenzamine and *Phentolamine* are non-selective antagonists of α-adrenoceptors (i.e. act equivalently at both α_1- and α_2-adrenoceptors). They are used in hypertensive episodes and during surgery in phaeochromocytoma.

β-ADRENOCEPTOR BLOCKING DRUGS

- A number of β-receptors classes have been identified, but with regard to pharmacology there are two which play significant roles.
- Under normal circumstances these are stimulated by adrenaline and noradrenaline.
  - β_1 receptors: Predominant effects are within cardiac and renal tissues.
    - Cardiac: Stimulation of the SA and AV nodes and myocytes leads to an increased heart rate via (chronotropy) and contractility (inotropy).
    - Renal: Stimulation leads to renin release.
  - β_2 receptors: Stimulation leads to smooth muscle relaxation, increases skeletal muscle contraction and increases glycogenolysis.
- Different β-blockers exhibit varying selectivity for the above receptors affecting their effect profile (see drug profiles below).
- The clinical effects and adverse effect profile is related to both direct and indirect actions of the drugs in addition to the pharmacokinetic profiles (discussed below).

Pharmacodynamics

- Competitively inhibit the β adrenoceptors reversing effects noted above.
  - Negative chronotropy and inotropy.
  - Reduced systemic blood pressure, thought to be due to suppressed renin production and reduction in cardiac output.
  - Increased smooth muscle tone (increasing in airway resistance, important in asthma/COPD).
  - Reduction in aqueous humour secretion in the eye (used in glaucoma).

Pharmacokinetics

- Distribution:
  - Water soluble: Atenolol, bisoprolol, sotalol (do not cross blood brain barrier).
  - Lipid soluble: Propranolol, carvedilol, metolprolol, timolol (increased CNS adverse effects).

Indications

- Cardiovascular:
  - Angina.
  - Heart failure (reduced sympathetic activity).
  - Post-myocardial infarction.
  - Supraventricular tachyarrhythmias.
- Neurological: Migraine prophylaxis.
- Ocular: Glaucoma.
- Other: Hyperthyroidism (symptomatic relief: e.g. tachycardia, palpitations), anxiety symptoms and portal hypertension.

Cautions and contraindications

- Cardiac: Uncontrolled HF, hypotension, bradycardia, AV blocks/disease.
- Respiratory: Asthma (contraindication), COPD (may be used with caution).
- Others: Abrupt withdrawal (up-regulation of receptors (see Ch. 3, Section 3.2) results in rebound sympathetic response with tachycardia), severe PVD and diabetes (may mask hypoglycaemia symptoms).

Adverse effects

- Cardiac: Heart failure, bradycardia, peripheral vasoconstriction (β_2 mediated).
- Respiratory: Bronchospasm.
- Others: Sleep disturbance (with lipid soluble forms), deterioration in glucose control in diabetes. May result in erectile dysfunction.

Important interactions

- Non-dihydropyridine calcium channel antagonists and class I antiarrhythmics can worsen reduced cardiac contractility and AV node conduction.

Drugs and practical prescribing

Examples

- Note ISA (intrinsic sympathomimetic activity) implies the drug blocks and stimulates β-receptors (i.e. partial agonist). These drugs tend to cause less bradycardia and peripheral vasoconstriction than other drugs.

Non-selective

- **Propranolol:** Available oral (including MR **Half/Inderal LA®**) and IV.
- **Acebutolol (Sectral®):** ISA (see above).
- **Carvedilol (Eucardic®):** Has additional α-blocking activity.
- **Labetolol (Trandate®):** Has additional α-blocking activity, safe in pregnancy.
  - Used in hypertension, including pregnancy-induced hypertension.
- **Nadolol (Corgard®).**
- **Oxprenolol** (MR -**Slow-Trasicor®**): ISA (see above).
- **Pindolol (Visken®):** ISA (see above).
- **Sotalol (Beta-Cardone®, Sotacor®):** Also Class III antiarrhythmic activity.
- **Timolol (Betim®).**

β₁ selective (relatively cardioselective)

- **Atenolol (Tenormin®).**
- **Bisoprolol (Cardicor®, Emcor®).**
- **Celiprolol (Celectol®):** ISA.
- **Esmolol (Brevibloc®):** Short acting, available IV. Used intraoperatively and for acute management of arrhythmias.
- **Metoprolol (Betaloc®):** Available oral and IV. May be used acutely post MI.
- **Nebivolol (Nebilet®):** Also exhibits NO mediated vasodilation.

5.5 ANTIHYPERTENSIVE AND RELATED MEDICATIONS

INITIATING ANTIHYPERTENSIVE MEDICATION

- Algorithms and guidelines are available regarding the appropriate initiation of antihypertensive medication.
- In the UK these guidelines have been produced in a collaboration between the British Hypertension Society and NICE (see MICRO-reference below).

MICRO-reference
National Institute for Health and Clinical Excellence. Hypertension: Quick reference guide. Clinical Guidance 127. London, UK: NICE, 2006. Available from: http://guidance.nice.org.uk/CG127/QuickRefGuide/pdf/English

CENTRALLY ACTING ANTIHYPERTENSIVES

- This class of antihypertensive is usually reserved for refractory hypertension or when other drug classes are contraindicated, though other indications exist (see individual drug profiles).

Pharmacodynamics

- These drugs induce vasodilation through reduced sympathetic arteriolar tone.
- This is mediated by reduced sympathetic outflow from higher CNS centres, including the vasopressor centres in the brainstem.
- Two predominant mechanisms exist:
  - Agonism of presynaptic α_2 receptors, reducing presynaptic Ca^{2+} levels required for noradrenaline release.
  - Agonism of I_1-imidazoline receptors which appears to reduce sympathetic outflow.
- **Methyldopa (Aldomet®):** Metabolites selectively stimulate central α_2-adrenoceptors.
- **Clonidine (Catapres®, Dixarit®):** Stimulates α_2-adrenoceptors, and may agonize at the imidazoline receptor.
- **Moxonidine (Physiotens®):** Has preferential binding at the imidazoline receptor. The minimal α_2-adrenoceptor binding results in an improved side-effect profile.

Indications

- Hypertension.
- **Clonidine:** Migraine, menopausal flushing and in critical care settings for sedation and acute pain.

Contraindications

- **Clonidine/moxonidine:** Cardiac conduction disorders, severe heart failure.
- **Methyldopa:** Depression, phaeochromocytoma, porphyria.

Cautions

- Clonidine and moxonidine:
  - Abrupt withdrawal results in rebound catecholamine release and a hypertensive crisis.
  - Arterial disease, including peripheral vascular disease and Raynaud's.
- History of depression (clonidine).

Adverse effects

- **Methyldopa:**
  - Psychological: Sedation, also depression and other neuropsychiatric effects.
  - Extrapyramidal effects: See Ch. 8, Section 8.4.
  - Hyperprolactinaemia: Rare.

- Blood disorders: Positive Coomb's test (in up to 20%), haemolytic anaemia, marrow suppression.
- Hypersensitivity, including drug-induced lupus, also myocarditis/pericarditis.
- **Clonidine:**
  - GI disturbance: Dry mouth, constipation, nausea/vomiting.
  - Neuropsychiatric effects: Sedation, depression, headache, paraesthesia.
  - Other: Bradyarrhythmia, AV block and hepatitis.
- **Moxonidine:**
  - Dry mouth, nausea/vomiting, diarrhoea, sedation.

Important interactions

- **Clonidine:**
  - Risk of withdrawal hypertensive crisis increased with β-adrenoceptor antagonists.
- **Methyldopa:**
  - Increased extrapyramidal effects with dopamine antagonists (e.g. antipsychotics).
- Avoid use with lithium (neurotoxicity) and MAOIs.

Special requirements

- FBC and LFT monitoring required for methyldopa.

VASODILATOR ANTIHYPERTENSIVES

- These agents produce arteriolar ± venous dilatation through smooth muscle relaxation reducing vascular resistance.
- They are generally reserved for resistant hypertension or when other agents are not appropriate or contraindicated.
- **Hydralazine (Apresoline®):**
  - Unknown mechanism of action resulting in direct arteriolar vasodilation and reduction in afterload.
  - Licensed in hypertension, but more commonly used in heart failure in conjunction with nitrates for combined veno- and arterio-dilation when ACE inhibitors are contraindicated.
- Associated with antinuclear antibody positive lupus-like syndrome (dose related).

MICRO-facts

Drug induced lupus

- An MRCP (Member of the Royal College of Physicians) exam favourite.
- More common causes include:
  - **Hydralazine, Isoniazid, Chlorpromazine, Quinidine, Phenytoin.**
- Further information about MRCP study available at: http://mrcpstudy.com/systemic-lupus-erythematosus/

- **Minoxidil (Loniten®):**
  - Sulphate metabolite activates K^+ channels stabilizing the smooth muscle membrane and resulting in significant arteriolar dilatation.
  - Used in hypertension with a β-blocker and diuretic to counter minoxidil's reflex tachycardia and fluid retention respectively.
  - Also leads to hypertrichosis (increased hair growth) and is available topically for male baldness (unsuitable for females).
- **Sodium nitroprusside:**
  - Nitric oxide release increases cellular concentrations of cGMP, preventing vascular smooth muscle contraction.
- Produces arteriolar and venous dilatation and is used intravenously in the acute management of severe resistant hypertension.

MICRO-print

Sodium nitroprusside and cyanide toxicity

Sodium nitroprusside can be broken down on exposure to UV light to release cyanide.

For this reason infusion bags containing sodium nitroprusside must be protected from light (patients on prolonged infusion may get cyanide poisoning).

- **Diazoxide (Eudemine®):** Similar to minoxidil and indicated in acute hypertensive crisis.
- PDE-5 inhibitors **(sildenafil [Revatio® Viagra®], tadalafil [Adcirca®])**.
  - These drugs increase cGMP levels in the pulmonary vasculature and corpus cavernosum of the penis resulting in smooth muscle relaxation.
  - This occurs through specific inhibition of cGMP breakdown by phosphodiesterase type 5 (PDE5).
  - They are indicated in pulmonary arterial hypertension and erectile dysfunction.
  - Cautioned with other vasodilator antihypertensives and nitrates (enhances hypotension).
- Endothelin-receptor antagonists:
  - Endothelin is potent vasoconstrictor with several receptor subtypes.
    - ET_A is found mainly in vascular smooth muscle.
    - ET_B is predominantly found in vascular endothelium.
    - Antagonism at these receptors prevents the endothelin mediated vasoconstriction.
  - **Ambrisentan (Volbris®)** is a selective ET_A inhibitor whereas **bosentan (Tracleer®)** binds to ET_A and ET_B and both are indicated in pulmonary hypertension.

Drugs and practical prescribing

- **Iloprost (Ventavis®):**
  - A synthetic analogue of prostacyclin (PGI_2), which is a potent systemic and pulmonary arteriolar vasodilator.
  - Used in pulmonary hypertension by inhalation of a nebulized solution.

DRUGS AFFECTING THE RENIN–ANGIOTENSIN SYSTEM

- Drugs in this class are widely used for a variety of indications due to their effects as described below.
- Three classes of drugs exist:
  - Angiotensin-converting enzyme inhibitors (ACEis) are commonly used.
  - Angiotensin II receptor blockers (ARB – also know as angiotensin II antagonists)
- Direct renin inhibitors, e.g. **Aliskiren (Rasilez®)** are rarely used.

Pharmacodynamics

Renin–Angiotensin–Aldosterone system

- Renin is produced by renal juxtaglomerular cells in response to reduced renal perfusion. This enzyme cleaves hepatically derived angiotensinogen to form angiotensin I.
- ACE produced largely in the pulmonary capillary beds cleaves angiotensin I to form angiotensin II. It also degrades bradykinin – a mild vasodilator.
- Angiotensin II (AII) has multiple effects which normally maintain blood pressure:
  - Potent vasoconstriction:
    - Arterial vasoconstriction increases systemic vascular resistance.
    - Glomerular efferent arteriolar constriction increasing renal filtration pressures
  - Stimulates aldosterone secretion from adrenal cortex.
  - Direct tubular Na^+ and fluid retention (with K^+ excretion).
  - Stimulates ADH release from the posterior pituitary.
- AII is also involved in ventricular remodeling after myocardial damage.

ACE inhibitors

- Binds to and inhibits angiotensin converting enzyme (ACE) reducing AII production and resulting in:
  - Reduction in blood pressure through:
    - Reduced systemic vascular resistance.
    - Reduced Na^+ and water retention.
    - Increased bradykinin levels (responsible for cough as adverse effect).
  - Decreased glomerular pressure:
    - Protective in hypertension.
    - Damaging if effective perfusion pressure not maintained (see below).
- Reduced ventricular remodeling and hypertrophy post MI.

ARBs

- Selective antagonists at angiotension II receptor (AT$_1$).
- Effects are similar to ACEis without the bradykinin mediated vasodilation and associated cough.

Indications

- Hypertension.
- Heart failure – shown to reduce mortality and improve symptoms.
- Diabetic nephropathy – shown to slow disease progression.
- Post MI – reduction in maladaptive cardiac remodeling.

Cautions and contraindications

- Cardiac: Severe aortic stenosis (risk of hypotension), hypertrophic cardiomyopathy, postural hypotension – especially first dose (increased with diuretics, dehydration).
- Anaphylactoid reaction: Angioedema, *erythema multiforme*.
- Renal and electrolyte: Risk of renal impairment (see MICRO-facts) and hyperkalaemia.

MICRO-facts

ACEis and renal function

- ACEi induces glomerular efferent arteriole vasodilation and consequently reduces renal filtration pressures.
- Any additional reduction in pre-glomerular pressures may lead to significant reduced renal filtration and result in renal failure.
- Caution is therefore required with hypovolaemia and diuretic use, renal artery stenosis (contraindicated in bilateral) and concomitant NSAID use (reduced prostaglandin mediated afferent arteriolar constriction). See Ch. 10, Section 10.2.

Adverse effects

- Cough: See above.
- Hyperkalaemia: See above.
- Angioedema: Accumulation of bradykinin.
- Orthostatic hypotension: See above.
- Renal failure: See MICRO-facts.
- Others: Pancreatitis, blood dyscrasias, cholestasis and altered LFTs.

Important interactions

- Diuretics: First-dose hypotension.
- NSAIDs: See MICRO-facts.
- Hyperkalaemia with other drugs raising potassium levels.

Drugs and practical prescribing

Examples

- Note: Some preparations available in combination with diuretics and other antihypertensives.

ACE inhibitors

- **Lisinopril (Zestril®):** 2.5–10 mg OD, oral. Max 35 mg (80 mg hypertension).
- **Perinodopril** (as salt) **Erbumine:** 2–8 mg oral, OD.
    - (as salt) **Arginine (Coversyl® Arginine):** 2.5–10 mg oral, OD.
        - More stable formulation – dose Erbumine 2 mg ≡ Arginine 2.5 mg
- **Ramipril (Tritace®):** Dose dependent on indication.
- Others: **Captopril, Cilazapril, Enalapril, Fosinopril, Imidapril, Moexipril, Quinapril, Trandolapril.**

ARBs

- **Candesartan (Amias®):** 8 mg (4 mg in HF) – 32 mg OD, oral.
- **Irbesartan (Aprovel®):** 150–300 mg, OD, oral.
- **Losartan (Cozaar®):** 50 mg (12.5 mg in HF) – 150 mg OD, oral.
- **Valsartan (Diovan®):** Dose dependent on indication.
- Others: **Azilsartan, Eprosartan, Olmesartan, Telmisartan.**

Special requirements

- U+E must be checked before initiation of ACEi and at routine follow-up after.
- First dose given at night to avoid symptomatic postural hypotension (may later be moved to morning).

5.6 ANTIANGINAL AND RELATED DRUGS

- These drugs include calcium channel blockers, nitrates and other related drugs.
- They act predominately through vasodilation with class related variance in arteriolar and venous dilation.
- Indications varying according to class due to the pharmacological characteristics.
- In addition to angina certain classes may also be used in hypertension and heart failure.

NITRATES

- These drugs lead to vascular smooth muscle relaxation.
    - Predominant effect is veno-dilatation, reducing cardiac preload and myocardial work.
    - Some arteriolar (including coronary) dilatation occurs reducing afterload.
    - Non-vascular effects may relieve symptoms in oesophageal, biliary and ureteric smooth muscle spasm.

- They are effective in angina and heart failure.
- The different pharmacokinetics profiles of the drugs and formulations available allow use in a variety of circumstances (see below).

Pharmacodynamics
- Nitrates are metabolized within smooth muscle cells to nitric oxide (NO).
- NO is an endogenous vasodilator produced in the endothelium.
- It achieves this effect by activating the enzyme guanylyl cyclase thereby increasing cytoplasmic concentrations of cGMP which reduces Ca^{2+} availability required for smooth muscle contraction.

Pharmacokinetics
- **Glyceryl trinitrate:**
    - Extensive first-pass metabolism, rapid action and metabolism (half-life ~3 min).
    - Sublingual/buccal/topical/IV administration avoids first-pass metabolism.
- **Isosorbide mononitrate:**
    - Oral bioavailability 100%, no first-pass metabolism. Half-life ~5 h.
- **Isosorbide dinitrate:**
    - Extensive first-pass metabolism, largely to isosorbide mononitrate.
    - Rapid absorption from buccal mucosa.

Indications
- Cardiac:
    - Angina (treatment and prophylaxis).
    - Congestive heart failure.
    - Heart failure in combination with hydralazine in patients with contra-indication to ACE inhibitors.
- Control of blood pressure during surgery.
- Other: Anal fissure (topically).

Contraindications
- Hypotension/volume depletion.
- Structural cardiac disease: Reduced or fixed cardiac output states including HCM, aortic stenosis, tamponade, constrictive pericarditis and mitral stenosis.
- Other: Intracranial hypertension.

Cautions
- Hypothyroidism, hypothermia.
- Avoid abrupt cessation (risk of rebound angina).
- Tolerance (see below).

Adverse effects

- Hypotension (including postural): Avoid use if systolic BP <90 mmHg.
- Headache: Vasodilatation of temporal and cerebral vessels.
- Others: Nausea, vomiting, flushing, rash.

Important interactions

- Hypotensive effects are enhanced by other antihypertensives and may result in syncope.

Examples

- **Glyceryl trinitrate (GTN)**
  - Sublingual:
    - Spray and tablets for treatment of angina as PRN use.
    - Longer acting buccal tablets are also available, **Suscard®**.
  - Transdermal: Prophylaxis of angina (must remove at night due to tolerance).
  - IV: Infusion for acute heart failure and control of angina/MI pain
    - Prescribe as 50 mg/50 mL, start at 1 mL/h and titrate to response.
- **Isosorbide dinitrate:** Occasionally used for prophylaxis and treatment of angina and LVF.
- **Isosorbide mononitrate.**
  - Normal release: Prescribed BD, oral at 0800 and 1400 (due to tolerance).
  - M/R: Approximate bioequivalence 40 mg M/R $\equiv$ 60 mg normal release.
  - Normally administered daily. At high dose may be administered twice daily to reduced peak effects. If so prescribe at 0800 and 1200 to reduce likelihood of tolerance.

MICRO-facts

Nitrates and tolerance

- Chronic administration results in tolerance (tachyphylaxis) and reduced effectiveness.
- The mechanism is unknown, but a nitrate free period (usually at night) allows a return of activity and must be considered in prophylactic prescriptions.

CALCIUM CHANNEL BLOCKERS (CCBs)

- This class of drugs is widely used and is broadly divided into two subclasses with differing pharmacology and resultant indications.

Pharmacodynamics

- CCBs bind to L-type calcium channels in cardiac and smooth muscle and therefore reduce calcium influx into cells. This results in:
  - Selective arteriolar smooth muscle relaxation of peripheral and coronary vessels.
  - Decreased myocardial contractility (negative chronotropy).
  - Sinoatrial node depression and reduced atrioventricular node conduction (negative inotropy).
- Calcium channel blockers have varying affinities for either cardiac or vascular smooth muscle which significantly alters their clinical actions:
- Dihydropyridines: e.g. **Amlodipine, nifedipine**.
  - Greater affinity for vascular smooth muscle and reduce systemic vascular resistance making them useful antihypertensives.
  - Cardiac effects minimal and diminished by reflex sympathetic mediated tachycardia which is unhelpful in reducing cardiac workload in angina.
- Non-dihydropyridines: e.g. **Verapamil** and **diltiazem**.
  - Greater affinity for myocytes and nodal tissue, resulting in negative ino/chronotropic effects reducing cardiac output.
  - Verapamil has highest cardioselectivity and its nodal conduction suppression makes it useful in supraventricular arrhythmias, though it may precipitate heart failure.
  - Diltiazem's effects lie between verapamil and the dihydropyridines. This is beneficial in angina as it does not precipitate reflex tachycardia like dihydropyridines.

MICRO-print
Nimodipine has high selectivity for smooth muscle in the cerebral vessels and is used to reduce neurological complications secondary to vasospasm leading to decreased cerebral perfusion following sub-arachnoid haemorrhage.

Indications

- Cardiac.
  - Hypertension.
  - Angina prophylaxis (dihydropyridines) or treatment (non-dihydropyridines).
  - Supraventricular tachyarrhythmias (non-dihydropyridines).
- Vascular: Raynaud's phenomenon (nifedipine).
- Neurological:
  - Prevention/treatment of ischaemic cerebral damage following SAH (nimodipine).
  - Prophylaxis of cluster headache (verapamil).

Drugs and practical prescribing

Cautions and contraindications

- Dihydropyridines: Cardiogenic shock, unstable angina, significant aortic stenosis.
- Non-dihydropyridines.
  - Severe hypotension/shock.
  - Severe left ventricular outflow obstruction (e.g. severe aortic stenosis).
  - Decompensated heart failure/cardiogenic shock.
  - AV block (contraindicated second/third-degree), sick sinus syndrome.
  - Concomitant beta-blocker use.

Adverse effects
Dihydropyridines

- Vasodilator effects: Flushing, headache, palpitations.
- Peripheral oedema: Common.
- Orthostatic hypotension.
- Others: Nausea, abdominal pain.

Non-dihydropyridines

- Cardiac: Bradycardia, atrioventricular block, hypotension.
- Others: Rashes (diltiazem), constipation (verapamil), vasodilatory effects (see above).

Important interactions

- Caution with the use of non-dihydropyridines with beta-blockers. May produce a profound reduction in cardiac contractility, especially verapamil.

Examples and dosing
Dihydropyridines

- **Amlodipine (Istin®):** 5–10 mg, OD, oral. Often used in acute hypertension.
- **Nifedipine:** Short acting. Standard release results in fluctuant blood pressure and reflex tachycardia.
  - MR preps include **Adalat® LA/Retard**.
- **Nimodipine** (see above).
- Others: **Felodipine (Plendil®), Isradipine (Prescal®), Lacidipine (Motens®), Lercanidipine (Zanidip®), Nicardipine (Cardene®)**.

Non-dihydropyridines

- **Diltiazem:** Standard release preparations are uncommonly used. Many M/R preparations available and more commonly used. Due to differences in bioavailability they should be prescribed by brand name (see other prescribing source).
- **Verapamil (Cordilox®, Securon®):** IV used for acute management of supraventricular arrhythmias.

OTHER ANTIANGINALS

Nicorandil (Ikorel®)

- Dual-mechanism vasodilatory action:
  - Potassium channel activator: Results in arterial (including coronary) dilatation and a reduction in cardiac afterload.
  - Nitrate effect reduces venous tone and decreases preload (see nitrates).
- Provides additional benefit in combination with other antianginals.
- Administration is 12 hourly in contrast to isosorbide mononitrate.

Ivabradine (Procoralan®)

- Reduces SA node activity and lowers heart rate.
- Licensed for:
  - Angina when beta-blockers contraindicated or ineffective as sole therapy.
  - Heart failure in combination with other treatments for patients with heart rate >75.

Ranolazine (Ranexa®)

- Shown in trials to improve symptomatic angina through unknown mechanism.
- Does not appear to alter heart rate, blood pressure, or vasodilation.
- Licensed in refractory angina.
- Multiple CYP3A4 mediated interactions.

5.7 ANTIPLATELET DRUGS

- In fast flowing arteries high shear forces reduce the ability of the clotting cascade to produce fibrin rich clots as seen in venous thrombosis.
- Endothelial damage exposes subendothelial collagen which results in the initiation, activation and recruitment of platelets which aggregate together bound by fibrinogen resulting in arterial thrombosis.
- Antiplatelet drugs decrease this effect through interference with the cellular mechanism which results in platelet rich thrombus.

ASPIRIN

- Low dose aspirin has been shown to be of benefit in secondary prevention of atherosclerotic diseases including MI, stroke and claudication.
- Clinical efficacy is not improved at higher doses, but adverse events are increased.
- It has also been shown to be of benefit if 300 mg is given acutely following a myocardial ischaemic event.

Drugs and practical prescribing

Pharmacodynamics

- Aspirin irreversibly inhibits cyclo-oxygenase (COX), an enzyme with two major isoforms (see NSAIDs) (see Ch. 10, Section 10.3).
- This enzyme is responsible for converting arachadonic acid into prostaglandin H2, a precursor of functional prostaglandins and thromboxane.
- Through COX-1 inhibition, aspirin inhibits platelet aggregation by altering balance between factors:
    - Inhibition of platelet thromboxane A_2 production, a potent vasoconstrictor and platelet aggregator.
    - Endothelial COX is minimally affected at low doses, so prostaglandin I_2 (PGI_2), a platelet disaggregator, is still produced.
- As COX inhibition is irreversible, the antiplatelet effect lasts for the lifespan of the platelet (5–9 days).
- COX inhibition also produces anti-inflammatory and mild analgesic effects, as well as adverse effects.

Indications

- Cardiovascular:
    - Secondary prevention of cardiac ischaemic or cerebrovascular events.
    - Following coronary artery bypass grafting.
    - Acute coronary syndromes (including prior to revascularization).
    - Acute stroke.
- Other: Mild/moderate pain and pyrexia, high dose (900 mg) may be effective in migraine.

Contraindications

- Use in children under age 16 (risk of Reye's syndrome, see below).
- Active peptic ulceration.
- Haemophilia and bleeding disorders.

Cautions

- Asthma (bronchospasm, not all asthmatics are sensitive) (see Ch. 10, Section 10.3).
- Uncontrolled hypertension.

Adverse effects

- See NSAIDs.

MICRO-facts

Reye's syndrome

Reye's syndrome is acute fatty liver and severe encephalopathy associated with aspirin use in children under 16 years of age. Treatment is supportive and recovery is usual, although severe brain injury or death may occur.

> **MICRO-print**
> **Aspirin overdose**
> Aspirin is weakly acidic, and in significant overdose, the treatment usually consists of IV fluid hydration, alkalinization of the urine (increases aspirin ionization decreasing renal tubular reabsorption; see Ch. 4, Section 4.3) and in severe cases dialysis.

Important interactions
- Increased bleeding risk with some antidepressants and anticoagulants.

Examples
- **Aspirin:**
  - Acutely post MI/stroke (once haemorrhagic cause excluded), 300 mg oral.
    – PR available if oral route not appropriate.
  - Prophylaxis of thrombotic cerebrovascular and cardiovascular disease – 75 mg, oral, OD.
  - Analgesia: 300–900 mg 4–6 hourly.

ADP ANTAGONISTS

Pharmacodynamics
- **Clopidogrel/prasugrel:**
  - Irreversibly inhibits binding of ADP to the platelet P2Y12 receptor.
  - This reduces activation and expression of the glycoprotein IIb/IIIa complex needed for platelet activation and aggregation.
  - Anti-platelet effect lasts for life span of the platelet.
- **Ticagrelor:**
  - Reversibly binds to P2Y12 ADP receptor at an allosteric site to ADP, preventing signal transduction and thus platelet aggregation.

Indications
- These drugs are most commonly used for a defined period following myocardial infarction for additive benefit in combination with aspirin.
- Licensing, duration and precise indication vary according to each drug.
- Clopidogrel is also licensed for monotherapy for prophylaxis and treatment of atherothrombotic events where aspirin in contraindicated or not tolerated.
- NICE recommends long-term **clopidogrel** following ischaemic stroke not associated with AF.

Contraindications
- Active bleeding or history of intracranial haemorrhage.

Drugs and practical prescribing

Cautions

- Cardiac conduction abnormalities.
- COPD (ticagrelor).

Adverse effects

- Bleeding: Normally stopped 7 days prior to surgery.
- Dyspneoa (**ticagrelor**): Mechanism unknown.

Examples and dosing

- **Clopidogrel (Plavix®):** 75 mg OD, oral (300 mg s/p MI).
- **Prasugrel (*Efient*®)** 60 mg stat then 10 mg OD.
- **Ticagrelor (Brilique®):** 180 mg stat, then 90 mg BD.

DIPYRIDAMOLE

- **Dipyridamole M/R** 200 mg BD, oral, is used in combination with aspirin in the long-term management of stroke, where clopidogrel is contraindicated.
- It may be used as monotherapy only if aspirin and clopidogrel are contraindicated.
- It produces antiplatelet effects by:
  - Inhibition of platelet phosphodiesterase reduces cAMP degradation and thus decreasing the responsiveness to ADP.
  - Inhibition of cellular adenosine uptake with a net effect of reduced platelet activation/aggregation.
- Due to above effects dipyridamole increases the effect and duration of adenosine if administered for dysrhythmias.

GLYCOPROTEIN IIB/IIIA INHIBITORS

- These drugs are for specialist use only to prevent defined ischaemic complications of PCI, and prevention of MI in unstable angina.
- They inhibit the glycoprotein IIb/IIIa complex on the surface of platelets, preventing platelet aggregation.
- **Abciximab** is a monoclonal antibody used in high risk patients undergoing percutaneous transluminal coronary intervention.
- **Eptifibatide** and **tirofiban** are used to prevent early myocardial infarction in patients with unstable angina or non-ST-segment-elevation myocardial infarction.

5.8 LIPID-LOWERING DRUGS

- Lipid-lowering drugs are used in the treatment of hypercholesterolaemia and in primary and secondary prevention of cardiovascular disease.

STATINS

- These drugs have been shown to improve mortality outcomes for cardio-vascular disease irrespective of initial cholesterol concentration in both secondary and primary prevention.

Pharmacodynamics

- Reversible competitive inhibition of hepatic HMG CoA reductase (3-hydroxy-3-methylglutaryl-coenzyme A) reduces cholesterol synthesis and increases clearance of low-density lipoprotein (LDL).
- The cholesterol-lowering effect of statins appears to be most significant at night, as this is when the majority of cholesterol synthesis occurs.
- Statins with short duration of action should therefore be administered at night.
- Small beneficial effect on high-density lipoprotein (HDL) and triglyceride levels.

Indications

- Hyperlipidaemia.
- Prevention of cardiovascular events:
  - Primary prevention in at risk individuals (diabetes mellitus, 10 year risk of cardiovascular event >20%).
  - Secondary prevention after cardiovascular events (MI, peripheral vascular occlusion, ischaemic stroke/TIA).

Contraindications

- Acute porphyria (except rosuvastatin).
- Severe liver disease.

Cautions

- Correct hypothyroidism prior to starting treatment (may correct lipid abnormalities).
- Liver disease.

Adverse effects

- Myopathy:
  - Myalgia is common, but true myositis is rare.
  - Rhabdomyolysis may occur.
  - Creatine kinase (CK) should be measured in symptomatic patients: discontinue statin if severe muscular symptoms and CK >5× upper limit of normal.
- Liver enzyme derangement/hepatic damage:
  - Mild derangement of liver enzymes common and not significant.
  - Jaundice/hepatitis occur rarely.

Important interactions

- Several important CYP450 mediated interactions noted which vary with each drug, and may require dose alteration.
- Common examples include:
  - Myopathy risk with antibiotics due to CYP450 inhibition (macrolides, fusidic acid, some antifungals, amiodarone and some calcium channel blockers).
  - Coumarins (including warfarin – increased effect).
- For full list see appropriate interactions source.

Examples and dosing

- **Atorvastatin (Lipitor®):** Long-acting metabolites, may be given in morning.
- **Simvastatin (Zocor®):** 10–80 mg, oral, nocte.
- **Rosuvastatin (Crestor®):** Long half-life, may be given in morning.
- Others: **Fluvastatin, Pravastatin** – both nocte administration.

Special requirements

- Monitor LFTs before treatment and after 3 and 12 months.
- Advise patients to report muscle pain/weakness.

FIBRATES

- These drugs activate the peroxisome proliferator activated receptor α (PPARα).
- The ultimate effect of this is:
  - Increased levels of HDL.
  - Increased lipolysis and elimination of triglyceride-rich particles.
  - Variable and less significant effect on LDL.
- They are normally used second-line behind statins, but may be indicated first-line in those with a serum-triglyceride concentration >10 mmol/L.
- In type 2 diabetes fibrates may be added to statins in patients with serum-triglyceride concentration >2.3 mmol/L.
- Significant adverse effects include a myositis-like syndrome, more common in renal impairment.
- Licensed examples: **Bezafibrate (Bezalip®), ciprofibrate, fenofibrate (Lipantil®), Supralip®160, gemfibrozil (Lopid®).**

EZETIMIBE

- **Ezetimibe (Ezetrol®)** selectively inhibits intestinal absorption of cholesterol via blockade of a sterol carrier protein.
- It does not affect absorption of triglycerides, bile acids or fat soluble vitamins.
- No beneficial effect on cardiovascular morbidity and mortality has yet been demonstrated.
- It is normally administered in combination with a statin.

BILE ACID SEQUESTRANTS

- These drugs bind to bile acids in the colon and interrupt the normal entero-hepatic circulation.
- This promotes hepatic conversion of cholesterol to bile acids and consequently reduces LDL-cholesterol levels.
- **Colesevelam, colestipol** and **colestyramine** are used in hypercholesterolaemia.
- **Colestyramine** is also used in pruritus and diarrhoea associated with biliary obstruction.

NICOTINIC ACID AND RELATED DRUGS

- **Nicotinic acid MR (Niaspan®)** inhibits the synthesis of cholesterol and triglycerides in addition to raising HDL levels. It is limited by its vasodilating and pruritus side effects.
- **Acipimox (Obetam®)** has fewer side effects, but is less effective.

OMEGA-3 FATTY ACIDS

- **Omega-3-acid ethyl esters (Omacor®)** and **Omega-3-marine triglycerides (Maxepa®)** reduce triglyceride levels and may be used as an alternative to fibrates.
- Little evidence for reduction in cardiovascular disease.

5.9 FIBRINOLYTIC DRUGS

- This class of drugs is used to break up thrombus within the vasculature.
- Licensing and evidence base varies between the drugs, but as a class they are used in the acute management of STEMI, thromboembolic disorders and acute ischaemic stroke.
- For STEMI, PCI is preferred, with fibrinolytics used if PCI cannot be achieved in time, or is contraindicated.
- Use should only be considered if benefits outweigh risks (see cautions/contraindications).
- They should all be administered as early as possible with highest benefits seen if given within 1 hour of symptoms.

Pharmacodynamics

- Fibrinolytics activate plasminogen to the active form, plasmin, an enzyme which degrades fibrin within clots and promotes reperfusion.
  - All drugs with the exception of streptokinase are direct plasminogen activators.
  - Streptokinase binds to plasminogen forming an activator-complex which activates remaining plasminogen.

Indications

- See above and individual drug profiles.

Cautions/contraindications

- Any condition where significant bleeding associated with use may be significant, e.g. recent surgery, trauma, aortic dissection, coagulation defects, history of CVA, uncontrolled hypertension.

Examples and dosing

- **Alteplase:** Only drug with license in ischaemic stroke. Also MI, PE.
- **Reteplase, Tenecteplase:** MI only.
- **Streptokinase:** Streptococcal protein. Immune reactions occur. Repeat administration may cause allergic reactions and loss of efficacy.
- **Urokinase:** Any VTE, also occlusive peripheral arterial disease and fibrin blocked intravenous catheters and cannulas.

5.10 ANTIFIBRINOLYTIC DRUGS

- **Tranexamic acid:**
  - Inhibits fibrinolysis.
  - Used to prevent bleeding or excessive fibrinolysis.
  - Common uses:
    - Management of surgical bleeding (common in orthopaedics).
    - Trauma with significant haemorrhage (reduction in all-cause mortality – CRASH 2 trial, see MICRO-print box).
    - Menorrhagia.

> **MICRO-reference**
> The CRASH 2 collaborators. The importance of early treatment with tranexamic acid in bleeding trauma patients: an exploratory analysis of the CRASH-2 randomised controlled trial. *The Lancet* 2011, 26; 377(9771): 1096–1101.

- Blood related products: Products available include factors III, VIIa, VIII, IX.
- The most common is **dried prothrombin complex (Beriplex®, Octaplex®):** contains factors IX, and variable amounts of II, VII, X. Commonly used for reversal of warfarin where there is significant bleeding.

6 Respiratory drugs

6.1 INHALED THERAPY

- Many drugs that are used for their effects in the lungs are delivered via the inhaled route. This aims to deliver drug directly to the airways, maximizing the local effects while minimizing systemic adverse effects.
- The bronchodilating effect of 2 mg of oral salbutamol may be achieved with 100 micrograms of inhaled drug.
- The amount of drug that reaches the airways is dependent on the type of inhaler and the technique of the user.
- With poor technique, the majority of the drug dose impacts on the oropharynx and may cause local adverse effects (e.g. oral candidiasis with inhaled corticosteroids) or is swallowed and absorbed systemically.
- Inhaler technique has a huge impact on the efficacy of inhaled drug therapy and should be checked regularly in all patients. Poor technique is the main cause of poorly controlled asthma.
- Inhaled drugs are also available in fixed-dose combinations (usually a long-acting beta-agonist and an inhaled corticosteroid), especially in the maintenance treatment of asthma and COPD.

Inhaler devices

- Metered dose inhaler (MDI):
    - A propellant gas is used to aerosolize the drug and produce a standard dose with each activation.
    - Requires coordination of activation and inhalation for aerosol particles to reach lower airways.
    - High velocity of aerosol particles means large proportion of drug impacts on oropharynx even with good technique.
    - Two 'puffs' usually prescribed with short-acting agents with the aim to get at least one good delivery of drug to the airways.
- MDI with spacer:
    - A large spacer chamber used with an MDI slows the velocity of aerosol particles and reduces the need to coordinate activation and inhalation.

- Accordingly, more drug is delivered to the airways with less deposited in the oropharynx.
  - As effective as a nebulizer in management of mild to moderate acute asthma.
- Breath actuated MDI:
  - Inhalation triggers activation of the device, removing the need for patient coordination.
  - As effective as MDIs, but more expensive.
- Dry-powder inhaler (DPI) (e.g. **Turbohaler, Accuhaler**):
  - Relies on inhalation of dry-powdered drug with no requirement for propellant.
  - Effective delivery requires a sufficient peak inspiratory flow rate.
  - The dose is usually delivered in a single 'puff'.
- With longer-acting agents, maximum dose of long-acting beta-agonist contained in each activation. Therefore, repeat dosing may increase adverse effects without increasing airway effects (e.g. salmeterol).

Nebulized therapy

- Conventional nebulizers use compressed air to aerosolize drug, which is then inhaled (may also be driven by high-flow oxygen).
- Little evidence to suggest any benefit over optimal inhaled therapy.

6.2 BRONCHODILATORS

BETA$_2$ AGONISTS

Pharmacodynamics

- Adrenoceptors are distributed throughout all body tissues and mediate the effects of endogenous catecholamines according to receptor affinities.
- Beta$_2$ adrenoceptors are present in smaller arteries and many smooth muscle groups, including in airway smooth muscle.
- Stimulation of beta$_2$ adrenoceptors results in smooth muscle relaxation and bronchodilatation.
- The beta$_2$ agonists are largely selective for beta$_2$ adrenoceptors, although some activation of beta$_1$ adrenoceptors will produce adverse effects.
- For example, beta$_1$ stimulation in cardiac tissue results in chronotropy (tachycardia) and inotropy.
- Beta$_2$ adrenoceptor activation also inhibits mast cell degranulation and microvascular leakage.

Pharmacokinetics

- Beta$_2$ agonists are usually administered via the inhaled route; oral and intravenous preparations of some agents are also available.

- Absorption:
  - Only ~10–20% of inhaled dose is deposited in the airways (most of the remainder is swallowed).
- Speed of onset varies between agents:
  - Salbutamol/terbutaline 5 min (inhaled) and 15 min (oral).
  - Formoterol 5 min (inhaled).
  - Salmeterol has a longer duration of onset, making it unsuitable as a 'reliever' agent.
- Elimination
  - Beta agonists are divided into short-acting beta agonists (SABA) and long-acting beta agonists (LABA) based on $t_{1/2}$ and duration of action:
    - SABA: **Salbutamol, terbutaline** (duration of action 4 and 6 h).
    - LABA: **Salmeterol, formoterol** (duration of action ~12 h) and bambuterol.
  - Ultra-long-acting: **Indaceterol** (duration of action >24 h allows once daily administration).

Indications

- Asthma and other causes of reversible airway obstruction (e.g. COPD).
- Premature labour (salbutamol and terbutaline licensed for use as tocolytics).

Cautions

- Hyperthyroidism (may stimulate thyroid).
- Cardiovascular disease (including arrhythmias, hypertension, QT-interval prolongation).

Adverse effects

- Tremor/cramps: Due to skeletal muscle beta-adrenoceptor activation.
- Tachycardia/palpitations: Secondary to cardiac $beta_1$ adrenoceptor activation.
- Hypokalaemia: Beta-adrenoceptor activation increases cellular uptake of potassium (may be used therapeutically in hyperkalaemia).

Important interactions

- Risk of hypokalaemia increased with concomitant administration of other agents that may precipitate hypokalaemia (e.g. diuretics, theophylline).

Examples

- **Salbutamol:** Dose inhaled 100–200 micrograms prn. Nebulized 2.5–5 mg QDS + prn.
  - **Ventolin®** (MDI, DPI, nebulized, oral, parenteral); **Airomir®, Salamol Easi-Breathe® (MDI); Asmasal Clickhaler®, Salbulin Novolizer® (DPI); Ventamax SR®** (oral)
- **Terbutaline: Bricanyl®** (DPI, nebulized, oral, parenteral)
  - With **budesonide** (see inhaled corticosteroids)
- **Bambuterol hydrochloride: Bambec®** (oral)

- **Salmeterol:** Dose 50 micrograms BD (2 puffs BD of MDI, 1 blister BD for DPI)
  - **Serevent Accuhaler/Diskhaler®** (DPI), **Serevent Evohaler®** (MDI)
  - With **fluticasone** (see inhaled corticosteroids)
- **Formoterol fumarate: Easyhaler Formoterol®**, **Oxis®**, **Foradil®** (DPI); **Altimos Modulite®** (MDI)
- **Indaceterol: Onbrez Breezhaler®** (DPI)

MUSCARINIC ANTAGONISTS

Pharmacodynamics

- The airways receive a rich parasympathetic innervation via the vagus nerve.
- Increased vagal discharge produces bronchoconstriction and mucus secretion via the action of acetylcholine on muscarinic cholinoceptors.
- Ipratropium bromide and tiotropium competitively inhibit the binding of acetylcholine to airway smooth muscle muscarinic receptors, causing bronchodilatation.
- The extent to which airway calibre is controlled by parasympathetic innervation varies between individuals and the bronchodilatory effects of the muscarinic antagonists are generally less than those seen with beta$_2$ agonists.

Indications

- **Ipratropium bromide:**
  - Reversible airway obstruction (including nebulized in acute asthma).
  - Rhinitis.
- **Tiotropium:** Maintenance therapy in COPD.
- **Glycopyrronium:** Maintenance therapy in COPD.
- Note: IV preparation available. Used for anticholinergic effects in anaesthesia, palliative care and hyperhidrosis.

Cautions

- Prostatic hyperplasia or bladder outflow obstruction (risk of urinary retention).
- Risk of angle-closure glaucoma.

Adverse effects

- Anti-muscarinic effects: See Chapter 8, Section 8.1.
- Others: Cough, headache, dizziness, atrial fibrillation, eye pain, rash.

Important interactions

- Concomitant use of other drugs with anti-muscarinic effects will increase anti-muscarinic adverse effects.
- Ipratropium bromide/tiotropium will antagonize the effects of cholinomimetic agents (pyridostigmine, galantamine etc.).
- GI effects of metoclopramide and domperidone reduced by anti-muscarinics.

Examples

- **Ipratropium bromide:** Dose MDI; 20 microgram 2 puffs QDS, Nebs; 500 micrograms QDS (Stop other inhaled anti-muscarinics while on nebulizer)
    - **Atrovent®** (MDI, nebulized); **Respontin®**, **Ipratropium Steri-Neb®** (nebulized)
- **Tiotropium: Spiriva®** (18 microgram DPI); **Spiriva Respimat®** (soft mist inhaler)
- **Glycopyrroinum: Seebri Breezhaler®** (DPI)

MICRO-print

Roflumilast

- **Roflumilast (*Daxas®*)** is a selective phosphodiesterase-4 (PDE4) inhibitor licensed for adjunctive maintenance treatment of severe COPD with bronchodilators.
- Inhibition of PDE4 results in increased levels of cellular cAMP, which reduces the release of pro-inflammatory cytokines and promotes smooth muscle relaxation.
- Contraindications: Active severe infection, severe immunological disease, active cancer, concomitant immunosuppressive therapy.

THEOPHYLLINE

- **Theophylline** is a member of the xanthine family (which also includes caffeine).
- **Aminophylline** is a water soluble form of theophylline, used for IV administration.

Pharmacodynamics

- Mechanism not fully understood.
- Produces bronchodilatation via several mechanisms (although respiratory stimulant effect may be the main mechanism of action).
    - PDE inhibitor especially PDE4 results in increased cellular levels of cAMP and cGMP (bronchodilatation) and reduced release of pro-inflammatory cytokines.
- Adenosine receptor antagonism prevents bronchoconstriction but is also responsible for the cardiac effects of theophylline (see below).

Pharmacokinetics

- Absorption:
    - Rapidly absorbed from the GI tract, good oral bioavailability.
    - Poor water solubility (aminophylline is a water soluble IV form).

- Metabolism:
  - Subject to hepatic enzyme interactions.
  - MR preparations maintain therapeutic plasma concentrations over periods of ~12 h.
- Therapeutic drug monitoring: See 'Special requirements' below.

Indications

- Reversible airway obstruction (starting at step 3/4 of BTS/SIGN guidelines; see reference below).
- Acute severe asthma (aminophylline).

Contraindications

- Acute porphyria.

Cautions

- Peptic ulceration.
- Cardiac arrhythmias/cardiac disease.
- Hyperthyroidism.
- Severe hypertension.
- Hepatic impairment.
- Risk of hypokalaemia.
- History of seizures/epilepsy.

Adverse effects

- Can occur at therapeutic plasma concentrations (10–20 mg/L), but more common when plasma levels >20 mg/L.
- Hypokalaemia: Especially if used concomitantly with $beta_2$ agonists.
- Others: Nausea, vomiting, tachycardia, arrhythmias, headache, insomnia, seizures.

Important interactions

- Plasma levels of theophylline are increased by smoking and alcohol consumption, as well as concomitant use of CYP450 enzyme inhibitors.
- Levels are reduced by concomitant use of CYP450 enzyme inducers.

Examples

- Dosing can be converted between aminophylline and theophylline using the following equivalence: oral aminophylline 225 mg ≡ 175 mg oral theophylline (i.e. 0.8 ratio).
- **Theophylline: Neulin SA®, Slo-Phyllin®, Uniphyllin Continus®** (modified-release)
- **Aminophylline: Phyllocontin Continus®** (modified release)
- Parenteral preparations available

Special requirements
- Aminophylline:
  - Administered as a loading dose, followed by a maintenance infusion.
  - In patients already taking theophylline, the loading dose of aminophylline is omitted and plasma levels must be checked before administration.
- Theophylline must be prescribed by brand as bioavailability can differ.

MICRO-monitoring

- Therapeutic drug monitoring: see Chapter 2, Section 2.4.
  - Therapeutic range: 10–20 mg/L.
  - Levels timing: Trough (pre-dose) level.
  - Follows first-order kinetics.
  - Approximately 3 days to steady state.

MICRO-print
Theophylline toxicity

- Toxicity may occur as a result of accumulation or deliberate overdose.
- Clinical features include severe vomiting, agitation, pupillary dilatation, arrhythmias (including ventricular arrhythmias), seizures, hyperglycaemia and significant hypokalaemia.
- Features of toxicity usually correlate to plasma-concentrations above 20 mg/L.
- Activated charcoal may be useful to prevent further GI absorption, especially following ingestion of modified-release preparations.
- Other treatment is supportive, including potassium replacement and management of seizures.

LEUKOTRIENE RECEPTOR ANTAGONISTS

- Leukotrienes are produced by the action of 5-lipoxygenase on arachidonic acid.
  - Arachidonic acid is the same precursor used in production of prostaglandins (see Ch. 10, Section 10.3).
- Leukotrienes are implicated in several stages of the pathogenesis of asthma (as well as other forms of chronic inflammation and anaphylaxis):
  - Leukotriene C_4 and D_4 (LTC_4, LTD_4) are potent bronchoconstrictors, and also act as stimulating cytokines for eosinophils.
  - Increase in airway microvascular leakage and mucus secretion.

Drugs and practical prescribing

Pharmacodynamics

- Leukotriene receptor antagonists bind to the leukotriene receptor $CysLT_1$ in the airways and on eosinophils and prevents activation by LTD_4.

Indications

- Prophylaxis of asthma (starting at step 3/4 of BTS/SIGN guidelines, see MICRO-print below).
- Relief of allergic rhinitis in individuals with asthma.

Adverse effects

- Hepatic impairment: Including hepatitis and elevated serum bilirubin.
- Churg-Strauss syndrome: Increased incidence noted, although may be due to subclinical disease becoming apparent following reduction in corticosteroid dose.
- Other: Headache, GI disturbance, bleeding disorders (including thrombocytopaenia).

Examples

- **Montelukast: Singulair®**, 10 mg, oral, nocte
- **Zafirlukast: Accolate®,** 20 mg, oral, BD

MICRO-print

Sodium cromoglicate and nedocromil sodium

- These agents may be used in the prophylaxis of asthma (they have no bronchodilatory action) but are now rarely prescribed due to the effectiveness of inhaled corticosteroids.
- Good safety records – may be used in children to prevent exercise-induced asthma.
- Act by inhibiting mast cells and other inflammatory cells, and so reducing the airway inflammatory response to allergens.
- Very poor oral bioavailability therefore delivered by MDI: *Intal®* **(sodium cromoglicate)** and *Tilade®* **(nedocromil sodium)**.
- Adverse effects include headache, cough, throat irritation and paradoxical bronchospasm.

6.3 INHALED CORTICOSTERIOIDS

- Corticosteriods have broad anti-inflammatory properties.
- Their beneficial effects in asthma and other causes of reversible airways obstruction stems from inhibition of inflammatory cytokine production and leukocyte function.

Pharmacodynamics

- Anti-inflammatory effects (see Ch. 9, Section 9.3) reduce tissue oedema and mucus hypersecretion that contribute to airway obstruction.
- Delivery via inhalation maximizes local effects within the lungs while minimising systemic effects.
- Beclometasone, budesonide and ciclesonide are equipotent whereas fluticasone and mometasone are roughly twice as potent.

Pharmacokinetics

- Efforts to increase local anti-inflammatory effects and minimize systemic absorption are focused on maximizing the amount of drug that reaches the lower airways (as opposed to being swallowed) and increasing the first-pass metabolism of any drug absorbed from the GI tract to inactive metabolites.
- Bronchial delivery:
  - Portion of drug that reaches the lungs usually 10–30%.
  - Up to 55% with **Qvar**® inhalers due to smaller particle size. Beclometasone delivered via Qvar which has a 2:1 bioequivalence compared to beclometasone delivery via non Qvar inhaler.

Indications

- Prophylaxis of asthma.
- COPD (some preparations).

Cautions

- Systemic infection.
- Potential for bronchospasm.

Adverse effects

- Systemic corticosteroid effects (see Ch. 9, Section 9.3):
  - Usually only occur at prolonged high doses, e.g. greater than 800 µg/day of beclometasone (or equivalent).
  - May be sufficient to cause adrenal suppression and a reduction in bone-mineral density.
- Local corticosteroid effects:
  - Oral candidiasis (risk reduced by using a spacer device and rinsing mouth with water after use).
  - Hoarseness.
  - Dysphonia.
- Other: Paradoxical bronchospasm.

Important interactions

- See Ch. 9, Section 9.3.

Drugs and practical prescribing

Examples

- Commonly used in combination inhalers with beta-agonists.
- **Beclometasone dipropionate: Clenil Modulite®, Asmabec®, Becodisks®** (DPI), **Qvar®** (MDI – approximately twice as efficacious as other delivery systems, as above.
- With **formoterol: Fostair®**
- **Budesonide: Easyhaler® Budesonide, Budelin Novolizer®, Pulmicort® Turbohaler®** (DPI)
- With **formoterol: Symbicort Turbohaler®**
- **Fluticasone propionate: Flixotide Accuhaler®** (DPI); **Flixotide Evohaler®** (MDI)
- With **salmeterol: Seretide Accuhaler®, Seretide Evohaler®**
- **Ciclesonide: Alvesco®** (MDI)
- **Mometasone furoate: Asmanex Twisthaler®** (DPI)

Special requirements

- Patients using prolonged high doses should be issued a steroid card as for systemic corticosteroid use.
- Inhaled corticosteroids (especially beclometasone) should be prescribed by brand name, as potency can differ markedly (see Qvar above).

6.4 OTHER RESPIRATORY MEDICATIONS

ANTIHISTAMINES (H$_1$ RECEPTOR ANTAGONISTS)

- Histamine is a locally acting amine hormone released as a result of mast cell degranulation in response to IgE and antigen binding.
- Local effects include vasodilatation and increased microvascular leakage, as well as chemo-attraction of other inflammatory cells.
- It forms an important part of the local and systemic inflammatory response and widespread release produces the clinical features of type I (IgE-mediated) hypersensitivity. For example:
  - Rash and urticaria
  - Bronchoconstriction and intestinal spasm
  - Widespread vasodilatation and capillary leakage in anaphylaxis
- All antihistamines have similar efficacy, though the sedative qualities of the older agents may be more beneficial in pruritus.

Pharmacodynamics

- Competitive H$_1$ receptor antagonists that prevent the effects of histamine binding.
- Also have anti-emetic effects, due in part to antagonism at vestibular histamine receptors.

Drugs and practical prescribing

- Blockade of H_1 receptors in the CNS results in neuronal inhibition. Older H_1 receptor antagonists have a marked sedative effect due to their ability to cross the blood-brain barrier.
- The H_1 receptor antagonists also act as antagonists for several other receptor families, accounting for some of their other effects:
  - Muscarinic receptors: Results in anti-muscarinic effects; may be useful in allergic rhinitis.
  - Alpha-adrenoceptors: May produce hypotension in some individuals.

Pharmacokinetics
- Older agents have a higher lipid solubility that allows them to cross blood-brain barrier (results in sedative effect).
- $t_{1/2}$ of older (sedating) agents ~4–6 h. Newer (non-sedating) agents generally $t_{1/2}$ 10–20 h (allows once-daily dosing).

Indications
- Symptomatic relief of allergy, including seasonal allergic rhinitis (hay fever) and urticaria/pruritis.
- Emergency treatment of anaphylaxis (e.g. chlorphenamine or promethazine use after adrenaline administration).

Cautions
- Risk of urinary retention (prostatic hyperplasia, bladder outflow obstruction).
- Risk of angle closure glaucoma.
- Gastric outlet obstruction.

Adverse effects
- Sedation: Significant drowsiness occurs with older agents (some useful as sleep aids). Newer agents much less sedating.
- Anti-muscarinic effects: See Ch. 8, Section 8.1. Less common with newer agents.

Important interactions
- Metabolism may be affected by inducer/inhibitors of CYP450 enzymes.
- Sedative effects of older agents increased with alcohol consumption.

Examples
Sedating
- **Hydroxyzine hydrochloride: Aterax®, Ucerax®**
- **Chlorphenamine: Piriton®** PO: 4 mg 4–6 hourly, IV/IM: 10 mg
- **Promethazine: Phenergan®** may be used as sedative
- **Clemastine: Tavegil®**
- **Cyproheptadine hydrochloride: Periactin®**

Drugs and practical prescribing

Non-sedating

- **Acrivastine: Benadryl®**
- **Cetirizine:** 10 mg, oral, OD
- **Levocetirizine: Xyzal®** isomer of ceterizine
- **Loratadine: Clarityn®:** 10 mg, oral, BD
- **Desloratadine: Neoclarityn®:** metabolite of loratidine
- **Fexofenadine: Telfast®**
- **Mizolastine: Mizollen®**
- **Bilastine: Ilaxten®**

Special requirements

- Sedative effects may impair ability to perform complex tasks (e.g. driving).

MUCOLYTICS

Pharmacodynamics

- Reduces the viscosity and volume of sputum in disorders where abnormal sputum production is characteristic (e.g. COPD, bronchiectasis).
- Mechanism of action believed to be due to altering the mucoprotein structures (reducing viscosity), as well as reducing goblet cell hyperplasia (reduces mucus secretion).

Indications

- Reduction in sputum viscosity (carbocisteine, mecysteine).
- Symptomatic treatment of COPD exacerbations (erdosteine).

Cautions

- History of peptic ulceration.

Adverse effects

- GI bleeding (due to disruption of gastric mucus lining).
- Hypersensitivity.
- Headache.
- GI disturbance (erdosteine).

Examples

- **Carbocisteine: Mucodyne®:** 750 mg TDS decreasing to 375 mg TDS as condition improves
- **Erdosteine: Erdotin®**
- **Mecysteine hydrochloride: Visclair®**

MICRO-references
Guidelines on the diagnosis and management of asthma and COPD (including guidance on inhaler devices)

Asthma
The British Thoracic Society and Scottish Intercollegiate Guidelines Network. *British Guideline on the Management of Asthma Quick Reference Guide.* London and Edinburgh, UK: BTS and SIGN, 2011. Available from: http://www.brit-thoracic.org.uk/Portals/0/Guidelines/AsthmaGuidelines/qrg101%202011.pdf

COPD
National Institute for Health and Clinical Excellence. *Management of chronic obstructive pulmonary disease in adults in primary and secondary care (partial update).* Clinical Guidance 101. London, UK: NICE, 2006. Available from: http://guidance.nice.org.uk/CG101

7 Gastrointestinal drugs

7.1 ACID SUPPRESSANT DRUGS

- These agents are commonly prescribed in conditions where control of gastric acid secretion is required, and have a number of indications.
- In certain cases they have the potential to mask symptoms or mistakenly be used to treat symptoms of underlying gastric malignancy.
- To avoid misdiagnosis, patients exhibiting 'red-flag' signs and symptoms should be referred for urgent endoscopy (see below).

MICRO-facts

Red flags and acid-suppressant drugs
- 'Alarm symptoms': bleeding, dysphagia, recurrent vomiting, and weight loss.
- Age >55 with treatment non-responsive new onset dysphagia.
- Non-responsive to treatment for 4 weeks: consider *H. pylori*.

MICRO-print
Gastric acid secretion
- Maintenance of gastric pH is controlled by H^+ ion secretion by the H^+/K^+ATPase (proton pump) of the parietal cells.
- It is a complex process involving negative feedback mechanisms and direct and indirect positive regulators.
- However, at the basal membrane of the parietal cells there are three direct mechanisms of activation which lead to luminal secretion of H^+ ions via the 'proton-pump':
    - Neuronal stimulation: Vagus nerve.
    - Histamine stimulation: At H_2 receptors.
- Hormone stimulation: Gastrin.

H$_2$ RECEPTOR ANTAGONISTS

- The first anti-secretory drugs developed. Now largely superseded by proton-pump inhibitors due to better adverse effect profile and fewer drug interactions.

Pharmacodynamics

- See MICRO-facts box 'Gastric acid secretion'.
- H$_2$ receptor antagonists are selective for H$_2$ receptors and competitively inhibit the binding of histamine, so reducing gastric acid secretion.

Indications

- Treatment of gastric and duodenal ulceration (including NSAID use and *H. pylori* infection related).
- Prevention of peptic ulceration (particularly in high risk patients including acute and chronic use of NSAIDs and corticosteroids).
- Symptomatic relief in gastro-oesophageal reflux disease (GORD).
- Where reduction in gastric acid is beneficial:
    - Prior to induction of anaesthesia.
    - Prophylaxis of stress ulceration in critically ill patients.

Cautions

- See red flags above.

Adverse effects

- GI: Diarrhoea may occur. Altered LFTs (rarely hepatic damage).
- Gynaecomastia (cimetidine only: due to interference with androgen metabolism).
- Cardiac arrhythmias (with rapid IV infusion).

Important interactions

- Cimetidine is a potent inhibitor of several CYP450 isoenzymes and is now rarely used.

Examples

- **Ranitidine: Zantac®** 150 mg BD (or 300 mg ON), oral. IV dose 50 mg TDS
- Others: **Cimetidine: Tagamet®, Famotidine, Nizatidine**

PROTON PUMP INHIBITORS (PPIs)

Pharmacodynamics

- See MICRO-facts 'Gastric acid secretion' above.
- PPIs bind to and irreversibly deactivate the parietal cell proton pump, preventing acid secretion into the gastric lumen.
- Irreversible binding to H$^+$/K$^+$ATPases means the inhibitory effect on acid secretion lasts for the life of the enzyme (~24 h), despite the drugs themselves having a short $t_{1/2}$.
- In ideal conditions, PPIs can reduce 24-hour acid secretion by up to 99%.

Indications

- Treatment of gastric and duodenal ulceration (including those caused by NSAID use and *H. pylori* infection).
- Prevention of peptic ulceration (particularly in high risk patients including acute and chronic use of NSAIDs and corticosteroids).
- Eradication of *H. pylori* (as part of combination therapy).
- Parenteral treatment of bleeding peptic ulcers following endoscopy (reduces re-bleeding in those at high risk).
- Symptomatic relief in gastro-oesophageal reflux disease (GORD) and chronic dyspepsia.
- Gastric acid suppression in Zollinger Ellison syndrome.
- Where reduction in gastric acid is beneficial:
  - Prior to induction of anaesthesia.
  - Prophylaxis of stress ulceration in critically ill patients.

Cautions

- See red flags above.

Adverse effects

- Gastrointestinal:
  - GI disturbances.
  - Gastric acid suppression increases susceptibility to GI infection, especially *C. difficile* colitis (consider stopping in presence of diarrhoea).
- Hyponatraemia.

Important interactions

- Omeprazole is a CYP450 enzyme inhibitor (other PPIs may also have similar effects) resulting in:
  - Reduced antiplatelet effect of clopidogrel due to impaired metabolism to its active metabolite.
  - Increased plasma concentrations of phenytoin, HIV protease inhibitors, cilostazol and warfarin (mild effect).

Examples

All PPIs are approximately efficacious at comparable doses. Choice may be considered on individual drug factors and cost (see below).

- **Omeprazole (Losec®):** Available as oral, IV and dispersible (**MUPS®**) (often clog NG tubes).
- **Lansoprazole (Zoton®):** Also available as **FasTab®**: Orodispersible and passes down NG tubes.
- **Esomeprazole (Ezomul®, Nexium®):** S-enantiomer of omeprazole, likely minimal clinical advantage over omeprazole.

Drugs and practical prescribing

- **Rabeprazole (Pariet®).**
- **Pantoprazole (Protium®)** mainly used in parenteral form.

Special requirements

- Rebound acid hyper-secretion may occur after cessation of long-term therapy; consider titrated dose reduction.

MICRO-print

Misoprostol

- Prostaglandins E_2 and I_2 inhibit gastric acid production by acting upon the parietal cells.
- They also have some positive effect on the non-parietal mucosal epithelium inducing protective mucus production.
- NSAIDs inhibit this prostaglandin secretion, resulting in a loss of mucosal protection and potential ulceration.
- Misoprostol is a synthetic prostaglandin E_1 analogue which inhibits acid secretion via its interaction with parietal cells, and helps maintain the mucus lining of the stomach.
- Used in the treatment/prophylaxis of peptic ulceration, including that caused by NSAIDs, and is available in combination products.
- Also used to stimulate termination in early pregnancy (thus contra-indicated in pregnancy).

7.2 DRUGS USED IN INFLAMMATORY BOWEL DISEASE (IBD)

- Management of inflammatory bowel disease relies on systemic and local immunosuppression.
- Medical management aims initially to reduce systemic adverse-effects through targeted medication delivery to the affected locations of the GI tract.
  - Differences therefore occur with pathology:
    - Ulcerative colitis (UC): Disease localized to colon.
    - Crohn's disease (CD): Diffuse GI tract disease.

STEP-WISE MANAGEMENT OF IBD

Step 1
- Local management:
  - 5-ASA and related medication (see below) used for local anti-inflammatory effect.
  - Special diets may be effective in Crohn's disease.

Step 2
- Steroids:
  - Local or systemic delivery dependent on pathology (see below). Often used in acute setting.
  - Steroid sparing agents e.g. azathioprine or 6-mercaptopurine (see Ch. 17, Section 17.1) may be considered for frequently relapsing disease.

Step 3
- Immunosuppressant agents: Infliximab or adalimumab (see Ch. 17, Section 17.1) may be considered for those refractory to conventional therapy.

Step 4
- Surgery:
  - UC: Total colectomy is deemed curative.
  - CD: Bowel resections and management of complex fistula disease may be required.

AMINOSALICYLATES

- These drugs use anti-inflammatory action of 5-aminosalicylate (5-ASA, mesalazine) for effect.
- This works via a topical action on the bowel mucosa.
- They are effective in mild UC and reduce remission rates when used for maintenance, but have limited effectiveness in small bowel CD.
- Due to extensive absorption in the small intestine after oral administration very little drug reaches the colon where it is required for UC or distal CD. Techniques to overcome this are discussed below.

Pharmacodynamics

- **5-aminosalicylate (5-ASA, mesalazine)** has numerous anti-inflammatory properties, including inhibition of prostaglandin and inflammatory cytokine synthesis and immune cell function.

Pharmacokinetics

- Three techniques are used to target delivery to affected areas of GI tract:
  1. Formulation techniques using mesalazine:
     - pH sensitive MR coatings:
       - Disintegrate at around pH 6–7 releasing drug in mid to terminal ileum and colon.
       - Brands are not bioequivalent so should prescribe by brand name. No one brand significantly better than other.
       - **Asacol® MR, Ipocol®, Mesren®, Mezavant® XL** (also has matrix release system), **Octasa®, Salofalk®.**
     - Continuous slow release: Throughout duodenum to rectum; **Pentasa®.**

2. Local release: variety of suppositories and enemas available for distal colonic disease.
3. Chemical modification of 5-ASA:
   - **Sulfasalazine, Salazopyrin®:** Bound with sulfapyridine (thought to have systemic anti-inflammatory/immunosuppressant activity, but also responsible for additional adverse effects). Cleaved by colonic bacteria releasing 5-ASA.
   - **Balsalazide, Colazide®** (a prodrug of 5-ASA) and **Olsalazine, Dipentium®** (a dimer of 5-ASA) are also cleaved by colonic bacteria releasing 5-ASA. They are associated with fewer side-effects than sulfasalazine.

Indications

- Treatment of ulcerative colitis and maintenance of remission
- Crohn's disease
- Rheumatoid arthritis (sulfasalazine)

Contraindications

- Salicylic acid hypersensitivity

Cautions

- Patients should report any bruising/bleeding or infective symptoms as they may represent development of a blood disorder (see below).

Adverse effects

- **Sulfasalazine** (related to sulfapyridine content):
  - Blood dyscrasias (including aplastic anaemia).
  - Oligo-/azoospermia.
  - Skin/bodily fluid discolouration, specifically a yellow-orange discolouration.
  - Crystalluria (may cause renal/bladder stones).
- All 5-ASAs:
  - Blood disorders (as above, though less common).
  - Hypersensitivity reactions (including pancreatitis, hepatitis, pneumonitis, myocarditis).

Important interactions

- Increased risk of leukopaenia when used concomitantly with azathioprine/6-mercaptopurine.

Examples

- See above.

Special requirements

- Monitor renal function.
- FBC if symptoms of blood dyscrasias.

CORTICOSTEROID PREPARATIONS

- Corticosteroids are frequently used in the management of inflammatory bowel disease:
  - In an acute flare high doses are used, including IV preparations in some hospitalized patients.
  - Typically corticosteroid maintenance is associated with more severe disease and poorer prognosis. Specialist advice should be sought.
- Local colonic delivery is preferable in distal disease to minimize systemic effects e.g. suppositories in proctitis or enemas in left sided disease.
- Some systemic absorption will occur. Pharmacology discussed under systemic preparations (see Ch. 9, Section 9.3).
- **Beclometasone dipropionate: Clipper®**, gastric-acid resistant MR tablets.
- **Budesonide:** Limited systemic bioavailability and reduced systemic adverse-effects.
- **Budenofalk®**, enteric coated capsules/granules; rectal foam.
- **Entocort®**, continuous release capsules; enema.
- **Hydrocortisone:** IV may be indicated (see above), also **Colifoam®**, rectal foam.
- **Prednisolone:** Tablets (high dose in acute cases – 40–60 mg OD), rectal foam.
- **Predsol®**, retention enema; suppositories.

7.3 OTHER GASTROINTESTINAL MEDICATIONS

LOPERAMIDE

Pharmacodynamics

- Agonist at opiate receptors in the bowel wall reducing peristaltic action and increasing bowel transit time.
- This increases resorption of water and electrolytes, reduces stool volume and increases solidity.
- No effect on opiate receptors outside of the gut, no analgesic effect or potential for misuse or addiction.

Pharmacokinetics

- Absorbed from GI tract, but extensive first-pass metabolism renders systemic bioavailability negligible.

Indications

- Acute diarrhoea (when infective cause excluded).
- Chronic diarrhoea in adults.

Contraindications

- Abdominal distension.
- Situations where inhibition of peristalsis is undesirable (e.g. ileus).
- Diarrhoea due to ulcerative colitis/antibiotic-associated colitis/bacterial gastroenteritis with systemic illness.

Adverse effects

- Abdominal cramping, bloating, paralytic ileus, urticaria and dizziness.

LAXATIVES

- Laxatives should be prescribed only when pathological causes of constipation have been excluded.
- The choice of laxative should take into account the nature of constipation (see MICRO-facts below).

MICRO-facts

Treatment of constipation

No hard and fast rules apply. Individual causes should be considered, and after physical examination the appropriate treatment option selected.

Treatment considerations and suggestions (see local policies)

Optimization of reversible causes should be attempted, i.e. stopping/ changing constipating drugs, correcting dehydration (oral or IV if required) and dietary fibre deficit.

- Rapid relief in acute constipation – in addition to above:
  - If hard stool in rectum/palpable descending colon – glycerol suppositories 4g, PR. Enema if inadequate response (e.g. sodium citrate/phosphate).
  - If above fails, consider fecal impaction: macrogol sachets 2–8 daily.
  - If slower response acceptable and no contraindications, consider stimulant e.g. docusate sodium 100 mg BD initially.
- Alterations in bowel transit time/peristalsis (increases water resorption from stool):
  - Common causes: Opioids, anti-muscarinic effects, hypothyroidism.
  - Treatments: Stimulation of peristalsis ± softening effect:
    - **Docusate sodium** 100 mg BD (up to 500 mg daily), also consider **senna/bisacodyl**. Other classes may be used additionally.
- Immobility/frailty: Encourage/support timely defecation. May need bulking agents/osmotic laxatives in addition to increased fluid intake.
- Obstruction/ileus: Constipation usually secondary to other pathology. Requires surgical support. IV fluids are important in maintaining hydration if vomiting/NBM. Stimulant and bulk forming laxatives are contraindicated.

Pharmacodynamics

- Simple laxatives exert their main effect by one of several mechanisms.
  - Individual agents may have more complex pharmacodynamics.
- Bulk forming: Non-absorbable compounds that draw water out of bowel wall to form bulky gel that distends bowel and increases peristalsis.
- Stimulant: Stimulation of the smooth muscle increases muscular activity and peristalsis. Bowel wall irritation also increases water and electrolyte secretion.
- Faecal softeners: Have a surfactant effect on stool that allows the penetration of water to enable softening.
- Osmotic:
  - Non-absorbable sugars or salts promote movement of water into the gut lumen.
  - Macrogols contain non-absorbable polyethylene glycols in an isotonic solution that are used for bowel cleansing without causing significant fluid or electrolyte shifts.
  - Newer agents act on gut wall receptors to relieve severe constipation (see MICRO-print box below).

Pharmacokinetics

- Local effect in bowel, no systemic absorption.
- Osmotic laxatives can produce an effect within 30 min after rectal administration (3 h after large oral doses).
- Stimulant laxatives also work quickly (2 h after rectal administration, 6–12 h after oral ingestion).

Indications

- Constipation (hard stools at lower frequency than is normal for patient), especially drug-induced.
- Bowel preparation before surgery or endoscopic procedures (bowel cleansing preparations).

Contraindications

- Intestinal obstruction (stimulant and bulk forming), acute surgical conditions, active severe colitis.

Cautions

- Severe dehydration, electrolyte disturbances (bowel cleansing preparations).

Adverse effects

- Abdominal bloating/cramps/distension (osmotic/stimulant laxatives): Due to digestion of non-absorbable sugars (occurs less with macrogols), and bowel wall stimulation with stimulant laxatives.

Drugs and practical prescribing

- Electrolyte imbalances:
  - Occur more frequently with salt-based osmotic laxatives (e.g. magnesium citrate) in renal impairment.
  - Significant fluid shifts in response to other osmotic laxatives may also result in electrolyte derangement.

Examples

- Bulk-forming: Ispaghula husk (**Fybogel®, Isogel®**)
- Stimulant: **Bisacodyl; docusate** (stimulant/softener) **Dioctyl®, Docusol®**; senna (**Senokot®); sodium picosulphate (Dulcolax® Pico)**
- Fecal softeners: Arachis oil enema, liquid paraffin
- Osmotic: Glycerol suppositories (some stimulant action); lactulose; macrogols **Movicol®**; magnesium salts; phosphate enemas; sodium citrate enemas; **Micralax®**
- Bowel cleansing preparations: Macrogols (**Klean-prep®, Moviprep®**); magnesium citrate (**Citramag®**); oral phosphates (**Osmoprep®**); sodium picosulphate with magnesium citrate (**Picolax®**)

Special requirements

- Bowel cleansing preparations are administered in a large volume of fluid (4 L over 2 h) and may be difficult for some patients to tolerate.

MICRO-print

Methylnaltrexone and prucalopride

- **Methylnaltrexone** is a peripheral opioid receptor antagonist that does not cross the blood brain barrier. It is used in the palliative care setting to relieve opioid-induced constipation that has not responded to other laxatives. It does not antagonize opioid effects in the CNS.
- **Prucalopride** is a serotonin 5-HT$_4$ receptor antagonist that acts as prokinetic and is licensed for the treatment of severe constipation in women who have failed to respond to prolonged treatment with other laxatives.

Both of the above agents are contraindicated in intestinal obstruction or acute surgical disorders.

MEBEVERINE AND ALVERINE

Pharmacodynamics

- Thought to produce gastrointestinal smooth muscle relaxation through a combination of local anti-muscarinic action and interference with calcium transport.
- Used as antispasmodic agents.

Indications
- Irritable bowel syndrome.
- Diverticular disease, painful dysmenorrhoea (alverine).

Contraindications
- Paralytic ileus.

Adverse effects
- Hypersensitivity.

Examples
- **Mebeverine (Colofac®, Colofac ®MR** [modified release])
- **Alverine (Spasmonal®)**

MICRO-print

Preparations for ano-rectal disorders
- Haemorrhoids
- Local anaesthetics and soothing preparations (e.g. bismuth, zinc oxide) in combination with corticosteroids are used for short term treatment of haemorrhoids:
  - **Anusol-HC®, Perinal®, Ultraproct®**.
- Anal fissures
  - Topical lignocaine may be used in the short term.
  - Glyceryl trinitrate (GTN) 0.4% ointment or diltiazem 2% cream may also be used for their smooth muscle relaxant effects.

ANTIMUSCARINIC ANTISPASMODICS

- The smooth muscle-relaxing effects of anti-muscarinics are utilized to reduce bowel spasm in disorders such as irritable bowel syndrome and diverticular disease.

Pharmacodynamics
- Atropine and dicycloverine readily cross the blood barrier which makes them likely to cause systemic antimuscarinic side effects (atropine is no longer used for this indication).
- Hyoscine butylbromide (and propatheline) do not cross the blood brain barrier and are poorly absorbed from the GI tract therefore their systemic anti-muscarinic effects are significantly less marked.

Indications
- Symptomatic relief in gastrointestinal and genitourinary muscle spasm.
- Reducing excessive respiratory secretions (hyoscine butylbromide).

Contraindications

- Myaesthenia gravis; prostatic hyperplasia, bladder outflow obstruction; gastric outlet obstruction; paralytic ileus.

Cautions, adverse effects, interactions

- See Ch. 8, Section 8.1.

Examples

- **Dicycloverine hydrochloride: Merbentyl®**
- **Propantheline bromide: Pro-Banthine®**
- **Hyoscine butylbromide: Buscopan®** (oral and parenteral)

MICRO-print

Ursodeoxycholic acid

- Naturally occurring bile salt used occasionally to (very slowly) dissolve cholesterol gallstones.
- Reduces the hepatic secretion of cholesterol thus increasing the concentration of bile salts and rendering the cholesterol more soluble.
- Ursodeoxycholic acid is now more frequently used in primary biliary cirrhosis where there is some evidence to suggest it improves liver biochemistry and histology.

7.4 ANTI-EMETIC DRUGS

PATHOPHYSIOLOGY OF NAUSEA AND VOMITING

- Vomiting is a complex process requiring co-ordination of cranial nerve and autonomic motor function and several secretomotor functions.
- The vomiting centre located in the medulla is responsible for co-ordination of these processes.
- There are numerous inputs to this centre, stimulation of which produces nausea and eventually vomiting:
- The chemoreceptor trigger zone (CTZ) is located in the floor of the fourth ventricle in the brain, and by virtue of lying outside the blood-brain barrier, can be stimulated by drugs and endogenous substances in the blood. Rich in dopamine D_2, opioid and serotonin 5-HT_3 receptors.
- Vestibular apparatus activation can result in motion sickness. Rich in histamine H_1 and dopamine D_2 receptors.
- The gut has many serotonin 5-HT_3 receptors, and activation by serotonin released as result of gut distension, drugs, radiotherapy, infectious organisms etc. is transmitted to the vomiting centre via the vagus nerve.

- Anti-emetic agents target several different receptor groups and are thus effective in different causes of nausea and vomiting.
- Knowledge of the likely cause of nausea and vomiting is therefore important in selecting the most appropriate drug.

5-HT$_3$ ANTAGONISTS

- Activation of 5-HT$_3$ receptors usually produces vagal stimulation which feeds into the vomiting center and into the CTZ itself.
- Activation of these will produce nausea and vomiting.

Pharmacodynamics

- Selective antagonists of serotonin 5-HT$_3$ receptors acting both peripherally (in the GI tract) and centrally (in the CTZ).
- Highly effective at relieving nausea and vomiting due to vagal stimulation or stimulation of the CTZ but not effective in vestibular nausea.
- Blockade of 5-HT$_3$ receptors in the GI tract prevents activation by serotonin, released by enterochromaffin cells as a result of numerous endogenous and exogenous factors (especially chemotherapy and other drugs).

Indications

- Treatment and prophylaxis of chemotherapy-induced nausea and vomiting.
- Treatment and prophylaxis of post-operative nausea and vomiting.

Cautions

- QT interval prolongation.
- Intestinal obstruction.

Adverse effects

- Constipation, other GI disturbances, headache, flushing, arrhythmias, chest pain/myocardial ischaemia, extrapyramidal effects and dizziness.

Important interactions

- Metabolism may be increased by inducers of CYP450 enzymes.

Examples

- **Ondansetron:** Tablets, oral solution, IV
- **Granisetron:** Tablets, IV
- **Palonosetron (Aloxi®)**

DOPAMINE ANTAGONISTS AS ANTI-EMETICS

Pharmacodynamics

- The phenothiazines (chlorpromazine, prochlorperazine, levomepromazine) and the butyrophenones (droperidol, haloperidol) are antipsychotic drugs that exert an anti-emetic effect through blockade of dopamine, histamine and muscarinic receptors in the CTZ and vestibular apparatus.

- Significant adverse effects result from interaction with a broad range of receptors:
  - Sedation occurs due to blockade of histamine H_1 receptors.
  - Dopamine antagonism may result in extra-pyramidal effects and hyperprolactinaemia.
  - Strong antimuscarinic effects frequently occur.
- Duration of use should be as short as possible to reduce potential motor effects associated with dopamine blockade (e.g. dyskinesias).

Indications

- Severe nausea and vomiting.
- Nausea due to vestibular dysfunction (prochlorperazine).
- Post-operative nausea and vomiting (PONV) (droperidol).

Cautions and contraindications, adverse effects, interactions and examples

- See Ch. 8, Section 8.4.

ANTIHISTAMINE ANTI-EMETICS

Pharmacodynamics

- Antagonism at CTZ and vestibular histamine H_1 receptors is thought to produce an anti-emetic effect.
- Muscarinic antagonism also contributes to effectiveness, particularly in ameliorating motion sickness, but also leads to adverse effects.

Indications

- Nausea and vomiting (including PONV).
- Vertigo and vestibular disorders.
- Motion sickness (cinnarizine).

Cautions and contraindications

- See Ch. 6, Section 6.4.

Cautions

- See Ch. 6, Section 6.4; severe heart failure (cyclizine).

Adverse effects

- See Ch. 6, Section 6.4; also hypotension (cyclizine).
- Antimuscarinic effects.
- Sedation.

Important interactions

- See Ch. 6, Section 6.4.

Examples

- **Cyclizine (Valoid®):** 50 mg TDS, PO/IV (IM also an option but is painful)

- **Cinnarizine (Stugaron®)**
- **Promethazine**

METOCLOPRAMIDE AND DOMPERIDONE

Pharmacodynamics

- Used for their potent anti-emetic effect, as well as their prokinetic effects (stimulate gastrointestinal motility):
  - Anti-emetic effect achieved through antagonism of dopamine D_2 receptors in the CTZ, as well as some effects on peripheral serotonin receptors in the gut.
  - Gut motility stimulation occurs via the peripheral cholinomimetic activity of metoclopramide and domperidone.
- The anti-dopaminergic effects of these agents may produce significant adverse effects:
  - Metoclopramide may cause extrapyramidal effects (see Ch. 8, Section 8.4); less likely with domperidone as it does not readily cross the blood-brain barrier.
  - Both agents may cause hyperprolactinaemia due to dopamine antagonism.

Indications

- Nausea and vomiting (particularly due to gastrointestinal disease).
- Migraine (metoclopramide).

Cautions and contraindications

- General: Elderly and young adults (15–19 yr – see below).
- GI: Gastrointestinal obstruction/perforation/haemorrhage; 3–4 days after GI surgery.
- Others: Cardiac conduction disturbances, epilepsy, phaeochromocytoma.

MICRO-facts

- Recent MHRA guidance has related domperidone to a small increased risk of serious ventricular arrhythmias and sudden cardiac death.
- Use is now limited to nausea and vomiting for the shortest period possible, at a maximum daily dosage of 30 mg.
- It is now contraindicated:
  - With conditions where cardiac conduction is, or could be impaired.
  - With underlying cardiac diseases such as congestive heart failure.
  - When receiving other medications known to prolong QT interval or potent CYP3A4 inhibitors.
  - With severe hepatic impairment.
- Similar restrictions have been advised for metoclopramide.
http://www.mhra.gov.uk/Safetyinformation/DrugSafetyUpdate/CON418518

Drugs and practical prescribing

Adverse effects

- Extrapyramidal effects: Common and dose limiting with metoclopramide (caution in young, teenagers and elderly. Limit use to 5 days and avoid high doses). Rare with domperidone.
- Hyperprolactinaemia: May result in amenorrhoea and galactorrhoea.
- Others: Neuroleptic malignant syndrome, QT interval prolongation and arrhythmias, GI disturbance.

Important interactions

- Prokinetic effects reduced by anti-muscarinics (e.g. hyoscine).
- Metoclopramide antagonizes anti-parkinsonian effects of dopamine agonists.
- Risk of ventricular arrhythmias when domperidone used concomitantly with erythromycin.

Examples

- **Metoclopramide (Maxalon®):** 10 mg TDS, PO/IV/IM (5 mg/5 mg oral solution available)
- **Domperidone (Motilium®):** 10–20 mg up to QDS (max 80 mg daily), tablets and suspension

---

MICRO-print

Neurokinin receptor antagonists

- The vomiting centre in the medulla has a rich supply of neurokinin-1 receptors, which when activated by substance P (a peptide neurotransmitter), invoke a vomiting reflex.
- The neurokinin receptor antagonist *aprepitant* (and parenteral preparation *fosaprepitant*) prevents the binding of substance P to neurokinin-1 receptors and their subsequent activation.
- They are licensed for use as an adjunct to dexamethasone and 5-HT$_3$ antagonists in the prevention of chemotherapy-induced nausea and vomiting.

7.5 ANTI-OBESITY DRUGS

- These drugs may be considered in addition to lifestyle changes in patients with:
  - BMI ≥30 Kg/m^2 if failed weight reduction after 3 months of diet and exercise.
  - BMI ≥28 Kg/m^2 if there are co-existing risk factors for cardiac disease.
- The only drug currently recommended is orlistat.

- Methylcellulose has been used to increase sensation of satiety despite limited evidence in the management of obesity.

> **MICRO-reference**
> National Institute for Health and Clinical Excellence. *Obesity*. Clinical Guidance 43. London, UK: NICE, 2006. Available from: http://guidance.nice.org.uk/CG43

ORLISTAT

- Specific inhibitor of gastric and pancreatic lipases decreasing hydrolysis of dietary fats.
- Dietary fat consequently passes through the GI tract rather than being broken down and absorbed.
- Impairs absorption of fat soluble vitamins (A, D, E, K).
- **Orlistat (Xenical®).**
- Over-the-counter preparations available at reduced dose.

Neurological medications

8.1 PARKINSON'S DISEASE AND OTHER MOVEMENT DISORDERS

GENERAL PRINCIPLES

- Pathogenesis of Parkinson's disease
  - Degeneration of the nigrostriatal neurones leads to:
    - Reduced inhibitory input in the basal ganglia mediated by the neurotransmitter dopamine.
    - Relative excess in excitatory input mediated by acetylcholine.

MICRO-fact

Parkinson plus syndromes
This term describes a number of neurodegenerative diseases which display clinical features similar to classic Parkinson's disease. The response to anti-parkinsonian medication, however, is variable and often limited depending on the pathology.

- Anti-parkinsonian medications:
  - Increase dopamine levels or agonise dopamine (specifically D2) receptors.
  - Decrease the cholinergic effect.
- Medications shouldn't be initiated until symptoms disrupt daily activities due to side effects and reduced efficacy associated with long-term use.
- Avoid abrupt cessation of medications as this may lead to neuroleptic malignant syndrome (see Section 8.4).
- Medications must always be prescribed on admission to hospital for both symptomatic relief and to avoid precipitating NMS.

- Avoid concurrent use of anti-dopaminergics which may antagonize therapeutic effects on anti-parkinsonian medications:
  - Antipsychotics:
    - Particularly 'typical' first generation with high D_2 antagonism (see below).
    - Under specialist supervision, drugs with lower anti-dopaminergic effects may be used for psychosis in PD, e.g. quetiapine.
  - **Metoclopramide** (domperidone is a safe alternative as it doesn't cross the blood-brain barrier).

MICRO-facts

Prescribing in Parkinson's disease
- Can be difficult but relies upon some basic principles.
- Avoid early use of levodopa due to long-term side effects and instead use antimuscarinics, dopamine agonists or monoamine oxidase inhibitors type B ($MAOI_B$) (see below).
- Use medications and the available formulations to 'work with' patients and the timing of their symptoms.
- In particular, some patients will suffer effects of excessive 'peaks and troughs' in drug levels (particularly with levodopa):
  - Avoiding peak associated side-effects (often dyskinesias):
    - Increase frequency of administration and decrease dose.
    - Use MR preparation.
  - Avoiding trough associated lack of efficacy ('off' periods):
    - Use MR preparations.
    - 'Booster' low dose fast acting levodopa preparations (e.g. **Madopar®** dispersible).
- Increase dopaminergic effects (dopamine agonists, COMT inhibitors and mono amine oxidase inhibitor Bs).

LEVODOPA (AND DOPA-DECARBOXYLASE INHIBITORS)

Pharmacodynamics

- Levodopa undergoes decarboxylation to form the active compound (dopamine).
- Unlike dopamine, levodopa can cross the blood brain barrier to enter the presynaptic striatal neurones within the basal ganglia.
- Selective peripheral breakdown of levodopa is prevented by the co-administration of 'dopa decarboxylase inhibitors'.
  - These drugs do not cross the blood brain barrier, and confer two benefits:
    - Reduction in peripheral side-effects of dopamine (nausea, vomiting, dysrhythmias).

- – Increase in cerebral drug delivery as more levodopa available in the blood.
- However, associated central side effects persist (psychological disturbance).

Indications

- Parkinson's disease
  - Used in elderly/frail and those with severe symptoms.
  - Avoid first-line in younger patients due to long-term effects (see below).

Contraindications

- Angle-closure glaucoma (pupillary dilation).
- Malignant melanoma, may reactivate.

Cautions

- Psychosis: especially if severe psychosis (see Section 8.4).
- Pulmonary or cardiovascular disease, particularly if at risk of arrhythmias (β receptor activity).
- Peptic ulcer disease.
- Hepatic and renal failure.
- Endocrine disorders (including hyperthyroidism, Cushing's syndrome, diabetes mellitus, osteomalacia, and phaeochromocytoma).

Adverse effects

- Nausea and vomiting:
  - Due to chemoreceptor trigger zone (CTZ) stimulation.
  - Use domperidone to treat as it doesn't cross the blood-brain barrier.
- Postural hypotension (usually resolves after treatment initiation).
- Psychological effects (e.g. psychosis, vivid dreams, hallucinations, confusion).
- Sudden onset somnolence necessitates caution with driving.
- Dyskinesias (see long term effects).

Important interactions

- MAOIs: Risk of hypertensive crisis – avoid for 2 weeks after stopping MAOIs.
- Antidopaminergics: Antagonistic effect – metoclopramide, antipsychotics.
- Antihypertensives: Actions potentiated. Increased risk of postural hypotension.

Examples

- **Co-beneldopa: Levodopa/benserazide**
  - Formulations: **Madopar®: Levodopa/benserazide.** Formulations:
    - Dispersible tablets (rapid action)
    - Capsules (standard preparation)
    - CR (controlled release) analogous to m/r
      - Note MR preparations have 30–50% decreased bioavailability.

- **Co-careldopa: Levodopa/carbidopa**
  - Full dopa-decarboxylation achieved at 70 mg carbidopa
    - Ensure this total is met in daily dosing using below preparations
  - Formulations: Expressed in mg as levodopa/carbidopa
    - Tablets: **Sinemet**®
    - Modified release: Reduced bioavailability (see above)
    - Intestinal gel
    - With **Entacapone: Stalevo**® for end-dose deterioration (see below)

Special requirements

- Pre-prescription advice
  - Patients and their families should be counselled about potential side effects, especially:
    - Daytime somnolence and driving.
    - Impulse control disorders such as pathological gambling, binge eating, hypersexuality.
- Long-term use: Associated with important considerations (see MICRO-facts box)
  - Dyskinesias:
    - In initial stages usually due to overtreatment.
    - In later stages may occur more frequently.
  - 'On-Off': throughout the day patients oscillate between being 'On' (functioning) and 'Off' (immobility).
    - These are believed to be due to fluctuations in plasma levodopa levels.
- 'End-of dose deterioration': Duration of action decreases with chronic administration.

DOPAMINE RECEPTOR AGONISTS

Pharmacodynamics

- Direct agonist at dopamine receptors.

Indications

- Parkinson's disease.
  - As initial therapy in younger patients.
    - Delaying use of levodopa may reduce dyskinesias associated with its long term use.
  - Reduce 'on-off' fluctuations when used in combination with levodopa.
  - Useful in advanced disease as they do not require intact striatal neurons for effect whereas levodopa must be converted to dopamine in the presynaptic terminals.
- Galactorrhoea and acromegaly: Ergot derivatives (**Bromocriptine, cabergoline**) suppress prolactin and growth hormone release.
- Restless legs: Moderate to severe.

Contraindications
- Ergot related: Can cause cardiac valvulopathy; exclude fibrosis before treatment.
- Pre-eclampsia.

Cautions
- As per levodopa.

Adverse effects
- Class specific: As per levodopa.
- Ergot related: Associated with fibrotic reactions (pulmonary, retroperitoneal, pericardial).

Important interactions
- Antidopaminergics: Antagonistic effect e.g. metoclopramide, antipsychotics.
- Antihypertensives: Actions potentiated. Increased risk of postural hypotension.

Examples
- **Pramipexole (Mirapexin®):** (where 88 micrograms base = 125 micrograms salt); MR preparations also available
- **Ropinirole (Adartel®, Requip®)**: MR preparation also available
- **Rotigotine (Neupro®)**: Available as patches
- **Apomorphine (APO-go®)**: See below
- Ergot drugs: **Bromocriptine, Cabergoline, Pergolide, Lisuride**

Special requirements
- Ergot related: Consider pre-prescriptive fibrotic checks and follow up.
- Examples include plain chest radiograph, echocardiogram, serum creatinine and clinical signs of fibrosis/heart failure.

MICRO-print

Apomorphine
- Potent D_1 and D_2 receptor agonist used in patients with refractory 'off' periods.
- Causes profound nausea and vomiting requiring pre-treatment with domperidone.
- Only available for SC infusion, and requires specialist input.

Drugs and practical prescribing

COMT INHIBITORS (CATECHOL-O-METHYL TRANSFERASE)

Pharmacodynamics

- Relatively specific central reduction of levodopa metabolism by COMT.
- Therefore increases the elimination half-life of levodopa.
- Also reduces 'Off' periods and allows reduced levodopa dose.

Indications

- Adjunct to levodopa in Parkinson's disease with 'end-of-dose' motor fluctuations.

Contraindications

- Neuroleptic malignant syndrome (see Section 8.4), phaeochromocytoma, traumatic rhabdomyolosis.
- Hepatic impairment.

Cautions

- Abrupt withdrawal (neuroleptic malignant syndrome).
- Ischaemic heart disease.

Adverse effects

- Increased levodopa side effects.
- Red-brown urine.
- Hepatitis (rare with entacapone, potentially fatal with tolcapone).

Important interactions

- As levodopa.

Examples

- **Entacapone (Comtess®):** Also available with co-careldopa (see above)
- **Tolcapone (Tasmar®):** Specialist prescription due to hepatitis risk

MAO$_B$ INHIBITORS (MONOAMINE OXIDASE)

Pharmacodynamics

- Selective MAO$_B$ inhibition raises dopamine levels by selectively reducing its metabolism.
- Does not affect other catecholamine levels like MAO$_A$ inhibition (see Section 8.2).

Indications

- Monotherapy in Parkinson's disease: **Selegiline** may delay need for levodopa therapy but increase mortality.
- Adjuvant therapy with levodopa to reduce 'end-of-dose' deterioration.

Cautions

- Abrupt withdrawal (neuroleptic malignant syndrome).

- Hepatic and renal impairment.
- Peptic ulceration.

Adverse effects
- Increased levodopa side effects.
- Hypertension/hypotension.
- Peptic ulceration.

Important interactions
- Risk of hypertension with some antidepressants.
- Risk of hypotension with MAOIs.

Examples
- **Rasagiline (Azilect®)**
- **Selegiline (Eldepryl®):** Dissolvable **Zelpar®** available

ANTIMUSCARINIC DRUGS

- Effective treatment of tremor, some improvement in rigidity.
- Limited improvement in bradykinesia.
- Mild symptom improvement in early Parkinson's disease.
- Side effects limit use (particularly in elderly who should be prescribed lower doses).

Pharmacodynamics
- In Parkinson's disease, the reduction in inhibitory dopamine leads to relative excess of cholinergic action within the striatum.
- Anti-muscarinics help restore this balance.

Indications
- Parkinson's disease.
- Drug induced parkinsonism (often used for antipsychotic side effects).
- Acute dystonia (procyclidine only).

Cautions
- Cardiovascular disease including hypertension.
- Hepatic and renal impairment.
- Prostatic hypertrophy.
- Angle closure glaucoma susceptibility (rare side effect).

Adverse effects
- Blurred vision (risk of angle closure glaucoma).
- Dry mouth.
- Urinary retention.
- Constipation.

- Tachycardia.
- Psychiatric effects including confusion, hallucinations, anxiety (particularly in elderly).

Important interactions

- Increased side effects with other medication with antimuscarinic action:
    - e.g. tricyclic antidepressants, antihistamines, MAOIs, antipsychotics.

Examples

- **Procyclidine**
- **Orphenadrine**
- **Trihexphenidyl**

AMANTADINE

- Weak dopamine agonist with mild antimuscarinic actions.
- Tolerance frequently develops.
- Indications:
    - Parkinson's disease (occasionally used as initial therapy).
    - Antiviral.
    - Post herpetic neuralgia.

MICRO-print

Other drugs used in movement disorders

- **Tetrabenazine** likely depletes synaptic dopamine levels. It is used in Huntington's chorea and tardive dyskinesia.
- **Piracetam** is used in myoclonus of cortical origin. Its mechanism is unknown.
- **Riluzole** is proposed to act by inhibiting glutamate processes. It is used to extend life in patients with amyotrophic lateral sclerosis.
- Botulinum toxin type a and b e.g. **Botox®, Dysport®**:
    - Neurotoxins produced by *Clostridium botulinum*.
    - Used medically they produce local muscle paralysis.
    - They are widely used for a variety of indications from focal spasticity to hyperhidrosis.
    - Most side effects are related to paralysis of affected or surrounding muscle groups.
    - May lead to distal muscles being affected and arrhythmias.

8.2 ANTIDEPRESSANT MEDICATION

GENERAL PRINCIPLES

- 'Monoamine' theory of depression:
    - Noradrenaline and serotonin depletion is known to cause depressive illness.

- Increasing their levels using medications is thought to reduce depressive symptoms though the mechanism is not well understood.
- Choice: Most antidepressants are equally efficacious, so base choice upon:
  - Patient tolerance.
  - Concomitant disease, see individual cautions and side effect profiles.
  - Current medications: Consider interactions.
  - Suicide risk: Toxicity of antidepressant in overdose.
  - Response to previous therapy.
- Management
  - Consider psychological therapy as a first line in mild depression.
  - Selective serotonin reuptake inhibitors (SSRIs) are considered first line pharmacological agents.
  - Antidepressants may take 2–4 weeks before clinical effect is seen.
  - Treatment should be continued for longer than 4 weeks before considering change of medication.
  - Failure to respond:
    - Consider increasing dose or changing medication
      - Second line: Lofepramine, moclobemide, and reboxetine.
      - Severe depression: Other tricyclics, venlafaxine.
    - Recurrent failure needs specialist intervention which may include MAOIs, augmenting medication (mood-stabilizers, antipsychotics) or ECT.
  - Anxiety/psychosis may feature in depression: However, avoid antipsychotics as they may mask an alternative diagnosis, seek specialist advice.
- Withdrawal: Withdrawal effects may occur:
  - Usually mild and self-limiting and vary with each drug class.
  - Higher risk for drugs with short half-lives (paroxetine/venlafaxine).
  - Consider gradual dose reduction over 1–6 months.
- Suicidal ideation
  - Antidepressant use has been linked with suicidal ideation particularly:
    - In early stages of medication.
    - In children/young adults and those with previous suicidal ideation.
  - If there is significant risk, observation of the patient should be considered.

SSRIs (SELECTIVE SEROTONIN REUPTAKE INHIBITORS)

- Equivalent efficacy to tricyclic antidepressants with increased safety in overdose.
- Reduced side effects compared to other antidepressants.

Pharmacodynamics

- SSRIs inhibit the reuptake of serotonin (5-HT) into the presynaptic terminal.
- This leads to increased serotonin levels in the synaptic cleft.

Indications

- Depressive illness.
- Obsessive compulsive disorder.
- Chronic anxiety (>4 weeks), including generalized anxiety disorder.
- Panic disorder, post-traumatic stress disorder, or social anxiety disorder (**sertraline, citalopram**).
- Bulimia nervosa (fluoxetine licensed).

Contraindications

- Manic phase of bipolar disorder.
- Concomitant administration with other drugs prolonging QT interval (citalopram/escitalopram only).

Cautions

- Hepatic and renal failure (consider dose reduction).
- Epilepsy (avoid if poorly controlled or if seizures develop).
- History of GI bleeding.
- History of mania.
- Cardiac disease, risk of QT prolongation (citalopram/escitalopram only).
- Diabetes mellitus (may alter blood glucose).
- Withdrawal effects: Variable GI disturbance, anxiety, sleep disturbance, electric shock sensations, headache.

Adverse effects

- Sedation and antimuscarinic side effects (less than TCAs).
- GI effects (common): Nausea, vomiting, dyspepsia, abdominal pain, diarrhoea/constipation.
- Hypersensitivity reactions.
- Hyponatraemia:
  - Possibly due to SIADH.
  - Consider if patients exhibit signs such as confusion or seizures.
- Others: Suicide risk, convulsions (see cautions), sleep disturbance/euphoria.

Important interactions

- MAOIs.
  - Risk of serotonin syndrome.
    - Tachycardia, hyperthermia, myoclonus, fits, coma, hyperreflexia.
  - Advise investigation into individual drugs profiles if changes are to be made.
- Anticonvulsants: May reduce seizure threshold.

Examples

- **Citalopram (Cipramil®):** Also available as oral drops
- **Escitalopram (Cipralex®):** Active enantiomer of citalopram
- **Fluoxetine (Prozac®):** Long half-life

- **Sertraline (Lustral®)**
- **Paroxetine (Seroxat®):** Short half-life – increased risk of withdrawal symptoms
- **Fluvoxamine maleate (Faverin®)**

Special requirements
- See notes above regarding withdrawal and suicidal ideation.

TRICYCLIC ANTIDEPRESSANTS (TCAs)

- Choice:
    - All TCAs have approximately equal efficacy so choice is determined by adverse effects.
    - The more sedating drugs are useful in agitated and anxious patients.
    - Less sedating drugs are useful in withdrawn patients.
- Dosing:
    - Higher doses are used in depression than for neuropathic pain.
    - Antidepressant effect unlikely to be seen at even higher neuropathic doses.

Pharmacodynamics
- TCAs inhibit the reuptake of serotonin (5-HT) and noradrenaline into the presynaptic terminal.
- This leads to increased levels of both serotonin and noradrenaline in the synaptic cleft.

Indications
- Depressive illness.
- Phobic and obsessional states (clomipramine).
- Nocturnal enuresis in children (imipramine).
- Neuropathic pain [unlicensed] (amitriptyline and nortriptyline).
- Migraine prophylaxis [unlicensed] (amitriptyline).

Contraindications
- Recent MI (cardiac risk – see adverse effects).
- Arrhythmias – particularly heart block.
- Manic phase on bipolar disorder.

Cautions
- Conditions predisposing to arrhythmias: cardiovascular, hyperthyroid.
- Conditions aggravated by anticholinergic effects.

Adverse effects
- Antimuscarinic side effects: May be marked.
- Cardiovascular: Arrhythmias, tachycardia, postural hypotension, ECG changes.
- CNS: Common including confusion, agitation/drowsiness, extrapyramidal symptoms.

Drugs and practical prescribing

- Hyponatraemia: Possibly due to SIADH, less frequent than with SSRIs.
- Others: Hyper/hypoglycaemia, hepatic and haematological reactions, suicide risk.

Important interactions

- Antiepileptics: Seizure threshold lowered.
- MAOIs: Risk of serotonin syndrome, as per SSRIs.

Examples

- More sedating drugs:
  - **Amitriptyline**
  - **Clomipramine, dosulepin, doxepin, trimipramine**
- Less sedating drugs:
  - **Imipramine, lofepramine,** and **nortriptyline**

MICRO-facts

Tricyclic antidepressant overdose

- All TCAs may lead to potentially fatal arrhythmias in overdose.
  - Amitriptyline and dosulepin are particularly dangerous.
  - Lofepramine is safer in overdose and has fewer adverse effects.
- Toxicity is predominately related to anti-cholinergic and autonomic effects.
- Common features include:
  - Cardiotoxicity with hypotension and arrhythmias.
    - ECG changes include prolongation of the PR, QRS and QT intervals, non-specific ST and T wave changes and AV block.
  - Metabolic acidosis.
  - Convulsions.
  - Serotonin syndrome (see SSRIs above).
- Initial treatment is supportive of symptoms with management of any associated hypoxaemia, hypotension or seizures.
- Acidosis should be treated initially with IV fluids and subsequently sodium bicarbonate if required.
- Any ECG changes and electrolyte abnormalities may require specific treatment.
- For more information see Toxbase.org or discuss with local poisons service.

RELATED NON-TRICYCLIC ANTIDEPRESSANTS

- **Trazodone**
  - Chemically unrelated to TCAs.

- Mechanism of action not fully understood.
  - Modulates a variety of serotonin receptors.
  - Likely noradrenaline effects of unknown origin.
- Sedative drug licensed in anxiety and depression.
- Other factors as per TCAs.
- **Mianserin** and **Mirtazapine**
  - Tetracyclic antidepressants.
    - Classified as noradrenergic and specific serotonergic antidepressant (NaSSA).
    - Modulates a variety of different serotonin receptors, increases noradrenaline levels by blocking central α_2 adrenoceptors and inhibiting reuptake.
  - Licensed in major depression, useful if sedation is required.
  - Associated with blood dyscrasias (mianserin more than mirtazapine).
    - Report signs of fever, sore throat, and stomatitis.
  - Mirtazepine available as oro-dispersible tablet, useful in dysphagia.

MONOAMINE-OXIDASE INHIBITORS (MAOIs)

- Rarely used class of drugs.
- Included in detail due to a number of significant side effects and potentially serious interactions with drugs and diet.

Pharmacodynamics

- MAOIs inhibit monoamine oxidase, reducing the breakdown of the amine neurotransmitters (serotonin, adrenaline, noradrenaline and dopamine).
- Two forms of MAO exist:
  - MAO-A: Serotonin, adrenaline, noradrenaline and dopamine.
  - MAO-B: Dopamine and phenylethylamine (used as anti-parkinsonian medications).
- Older irreversible, non-selective inhibitors are rarely used due to a high side effect profile and dangerous interactions (see below).
- Newer reversible MAO-A selective inhibitors have fewer side effects and interactions and have increased drug use within the class.

Indications

- Major depression, usually when other agents have failed.
- Social anxiety disorder (moclobemide only).

Contraindications

- Class specific: Manic phase of bipolar disorder, phaeochromocytoma.
- Others: Cerebrovascular disease with non-selective irreversible drugs.

Drugs and practical prescribing

Cautions

- Multiple interactions and dietary restrictions (see interactions and MICRO-facts box).
- Cardiovascular disease: Risk of postural hypotension and hypertension.
- Withdrawal: Agitation, cerebellar signs, hallucinations/delusions and vivid dreams (withdraw slowly if possible).
- Hepatic disease.
- Epilepsy.

Adverse effects

- Cardiovascular: Postural hypotension and dizziness (common).
- Anticholinergic effects: See antimuscarinic drugs above.
- Others: Headache, weight gain, sexual disturbances, oedema, drowsiness, myoclonus.
- Blood: Blood dyscrasias (leucopenia).
- Rare but serious: Hepatotoxicity, hypertensive crisis, serotonin syndrome, psychotic reactions, convulsions, peripheral neuropathy (possibly due to pyridoxine deficiency).

Important interactions

- Amine containing products: Serious risk, see MICRO-facts box.
- Other antidepressants: Including **bupropion** for smoking cessation (see SSRIs above).
- Antihypertensives: Enhanced hypotensive effect.
- Antiepileptics: Antagonism of effect.
- Analgesics:
  - Opioids: CNS excitation/depression, hypo/hypertension due to competition for metabolism leading to increased levels.
  - Nefopam.
- **Pethidine:** Hyperpyrexia and cardiovascular instability (probably due to reduced 5-HT re-uptake and reduced MAOI mediated breakdown).

MICRO-facts

MAOI interactions with amines

- Any amine product normally broken down by MAO directly or indirectly leads to noradrenaline release causing potentially fatal hypertensive and hyperthermic reactions.

continued...

continued...

- Products to avoid:
  - Direct sympathomimetics: e.g. decongestant medication.
  - Indirect sympathomimetics: including vasopressors.
    - Tyramine – cheese
    - Dopamine – broad bean, levodopa
    - Other amines – some fermented products (yoghurt, beer, wine)

Examples

- Non-selective irreversible MAOIs: Specialist only: **Phenelzine, isocarboxazid, tranylcypromine**
- Reversible (selective) inhibitors of MAO-A (RIMA)
- **Moclobemide**

Special requirements

- Dietary restriction and interactions as above.

OTHER ANTIDEPRESSANTS

Serotonin–noradrenaline reuptake inhibitors (SNRIs)

- **Venlafaxine (Efexor®) XL**
  - Potent SNRI.
  - May have greater efficacy than other antidepressants at higher doses where noradrenaline effects more prominent.
  - Indicated in major depression and generalized anxiety disorder.
  - Associated with cardiac toxicity and hypertension and requires initial investigation of ECG and BP and routine follow-up.
  - Risk of withdrawal due to short half-life.
  - Other cautions and considerations as per SSRIs (see SSRIs above).
- **Duloxetine (Cymbalta®, Yentreve®)**
  - SNRI licensed for:
    - Major depressive disorder and generalized anxiety disorder.
    - Diabetic neuropathy.
    - Stress urinary incontinence.
  - Other cautions and considerations as per SSRIs (see SSRIs above).

Noradrenaline reuptake inhibitors (NRIs)

- **Reboxetine (Edronax®):**
  - No serotonergic effects in contrast to most other antidepressants.
  - Licensed for major depression.

> **MICRO-print**
> **Uncommon antidepressants**
> - **Agomelatine:** Melatonin receptor agonist and a selective serotonin-receptor antagonist.
> - **Flupentixol:** Anti-psychotic with antidepressant properties at low doses.
> - **Tryptophan:** Adjuvant antidepressant for specialist use, associated with eosinophilia-myalgia syndrome.

8.3 ANTIEPILEPTIC MEDICATIONS

GENERAL PRINCIPLES

Mechanism of action of antiepileptic medications

- The physiological mechanisms of these medications are poorly understood.
- They are thought to block repetitive neuronal firing through the following mechanisms:
  - Neurotransmitter balance:
    - Reduction of excitatory neurotransmitter glutamate or interactions with its NMDA receptor.
    - Enhancement of inhibitory neurotransmitter GABA (increasing intra-neuronal chloride ion influx).
  - Cellular level activity:
    - Neuronal Na^+ channel inhibition, preferential binding of closed Na^+ channels prolonging inactivated state.
    - Reduced likelihood of repetitive firing, while normal cerebral low frequency firing unaffected.
    - Inhibition of thalamic T-type Ca^{2+} channels reducing spikes of activity associated with absence seizures.

Choice

- Based upon seizure type, clinical effectiveness and patient tolerance.
- Monotherapy is ideal to reduce side-effect potential.
- Doses are titrated to clinical response.
  - Drug plasma levels are only useful as an indicator of concordance and for assessing toxicity.
  - Dose adjustment is predominately lead by clinical response to therapy.
- Second line medications are used if there is treatment failure or intolerance.
- Adjuvant therapy should only be considered if monotherapy has failed to control seizures.
- It may not increase efficacy and increase adverse effects.

MICRO-facts

Antiepileptic choice

- Focal seizures:
  - First line: Carbamazepine, Lamotrigine
  - Second line: Levetiracetam, Oxcarbazepine, Sodium Valproate
- Generalized tonic-clonic seizures:
  - First line: Sodium Valproate, Lamotrigine
  - Second line: Carbamazepine, Oxcarbazepine
- Absence seizures:
  - First line: Sodium Valproate, Ethosuximide
  - Second line: Lamotrigine
- Myoclonic seizures:
  - First line: Sodium Valproate
  - Second line: Levetiracetam, Topiramate

MICRO-reference

National Institute for Health and Clinical Excellence. *Epilepsy*. Clinical Guidance 137. London, UK: NICE, 2012. Available from: http://guidance.nice.org.uk/CG137

Pregnancy

- Antiepileptics (particularly phenytoin and valproate) are associated with teratogenicity.
- Specialist advice should be sought.
- Prescribe folic acid (5 mg daily) prior to conception.

Withdrawal

- Abrupt withdrawal may precipitate rebound seizures; however controlled withdrawal may be attempted for patients who are seizure free for several years.

Interactions

- A common issue with many antiepileptics and should be considered during prescribing.

Driving

- Driving permitted (not heavy goods/public service vehicles) if seizure free for a year, or established sleep only seizures without awake attacks for 3 years.

> **MICRO-reference**
> Current DVLA medical guidance. https://www.gov.uk/
> current-medical-guidelines-dvla-guidance-for-professionals

CARBAMAZEPINE AND RELATED ANTIEPILEPTIC DRUGS

Pharmacodynamics

- Na⁺ channel blocking (see mechanism of action above).

Indications

- Partial (focal) seizures ± secondary generalization (eslicarbazepine licensed as adjuvant only).
- Generalized tonic-clonic seizures (carbamazepine only).
- Trigeminal neuralgia (carbamazepine only).
- Prophylaxis of bipolar disorder unresponsive to lithium (carbamazepine only).

Contraindications

- Class specific AV conduction abnormalities (unless paced).
- History of bone-marrow depression.

Cautions

- Cardiac disease (see contraindications).
- Blood, hepatic and skin disorders (see adverse effects).
- History of antiepileptic hypersensitivity syndrome (see below).

Adverse effects

- GI: Nausea and vomiting, occasionally diarrhoea.
- Neurological: Dizziness, ataxia, confusion, rarely nystagmus, peripheral neuropathy.
- Cardiovascular: AV block with syncope, exacerbation coronary artery disease.
- Hepatic: Rarely hepatitis, jaundice.
- Blood: Bone marrow suppression.
- Skin: Pigmentation alteration, rash, purpura, Stevens-Johnson syndrome.
- Others: Hyponatraemia, galactorrhoea, hypersensitivity reactions, anticholinergic effects.

Important interactions

- Due to hepatic enzyme induction, multiple interactions may occur.
- Note carbamazepine is an 'auto-inducer' and induces its own metabolism.

Examples
- **Carbamazepine (Tegretol®)** 200 mg–1.2 g, oral, in divided doses
  - MR preparation available for peak dose toxicity: 15% reduction in bioavailability compared to normal release
  - Liquid, chewable tablet and suppositories also available
- **Eslicarbazepine (Zebinex®)**
- **Oxcarbazepine (Trileptal®)**

Special requirements
- For carbamazepine and oxcarbazepine patients should be advised on recognition of signs of blood, liver, or skin disorders and to seek immediate medical attention if symptoms such as fever, rash (AHS – see MICRO-print box), mouth ulcers, bruising, or bleeding (blood dyscrasias) develop.

MICRO-print
Anticonvulsant hypersensitivity syndrome (AHS)
- This is a condition characterized by the triad of rash, fever and end-organ involvement (often hepatic).
- It is most commonly reported with phenytoin, carbamazepine and phenobarbitone, but has also been reported with other anticonvulsants including lamotrigine.
- It may have delayed onset after treatment initiation, and can be serious and even fatal. Suspicion should rouse a full medical assessment.
- IV corticosteroids are usually required for full recovery.

Bohan, KH et al. Anticonvulsant hypersensitivity syndrome: Implications for pharmaceutical care. *Pharmacotherapy* 2007; 27(10): 1425–1439.
Blondin, NA et al. A case of lamotrigine-associated anticonvulsant hypersensitivity syndrome. *Primary Care Companion to the Journal of Clinical Psychiatry* 2008; 10(3): 249–250.

SODIUM VALPROATE

Pharmacodynamics
- Likely effect is due to Na^+ channel blocking and GABA potentiation (see mechanism of action above).

Pharmacokinetics
- Absorption: 95–100% bioavailability. Use equivalent dose PO/IV.

Indications

- All forms of epilepsy.
- Bipolar disorder (unlicensed, also see Valproic acid below).

Contraindications

- Active liver disease or personal/family history of severe hepatic dysfunction.

Cautions

- Liver toxicity: monitor liver function (including PT).
- Renal impairment.
- Pregnancy (teratogenicity).

Adverse effects

- Gastrointestinal: Nausea, vomiting (reduced by use of EC formulation).
- Neurological: Ataxia, tremor, incoordination.
- Others: Hair loss, rarely: liver dysfunction, rashes, blood dyscrasias, pancreatitis, menstrual disturbance.

Important interactions

- Antidepressants and antipsychotics may lower seizure threshold.
- Important interactions with many other antiepileptics.

Examples and dosing

- **Sodium valproate (Epilim®):** 600 mg–2.5 g daily in 2–3 divided doses.
  - Available as crushable tablets, enteric coated tablets (e/c), m/r **Epilim Chrono®**, liquid/syrups, granules (for mixing with food), IV.
  - All considered to have equivalent bioavailability, no dose change required.
- **Valproic acid** (as semi-sodium salt) (**Depakote® Convulex®**).
  - Same active ingredient as above, branded as different chemical formulation.
- Licensed for manic episodes associated with bipolar disorder.

Special requirements

- Advise patients need to be aware of signs of blood and hepatic disorders and pancreatitis.

PHENYTOIN

Pharmacodynamics

- Stabilizes seizure activity rather than raising seizure threshold.
- Acts by neuronal Na^+ channel inhibition (see mechanism of action above).

Pharmacokinetics

- Absorption: Highly absorbed. Formulation variable (see special requirements).

- Metabolism: Hydroxylated in the liver. Potential saturation of this system leads to zero order kinetics and affects dosing requirements. (See Ch. 1, and Ch. 2, Sections 2.2, 2.3, 2.4)
- Protein binding: Highly protein bound (see MICRO-facts box).
- Distribution/elimination: Mean half-life is 22 hours (dependant on metabolism), steady state achieved in 7–10 days.

Indications

- All forms of epilepsy except absence seizures.
- Status epilepticus (see below).
- Trigeminal neuralgia if carbamazepine inappropriate.

Contraindications

- Phenytoin hypersensitivity, AHS (see MICRO-facts above).

Cautions

- Hepatic impairment.

Adverse effects

- Gastrointestinal: Nausea and vomiting, gingival hyperplasia.
- Dermatological: Rash (AHS), Stevens-Johnson syndrome, toxic epidermal necrolysis.
- Blood dyscrasias.
- Metabolic: May reduce vitamin D levels, consider supplementation.
- Toxicity: Nystagmus, diplopia, slurred speech, ataxia, confusion, hyperglycaemia.

Important interactions

- Enzyme induction:
  - Multiple interactions, including increased metabolism of warfarin, oestrogen and progesterone.
  - Phenytoin metabolism itself is increased by other drugs.
- Anti-epileptic effect reduced by antidepressants and antipsychotics.

Examples

- **Phenytoin (Epanutin®):** 150–500 mg, oral, in 1–2 divided doses.
  - Alter maintenance dose by 25–50 mg only due to pharmacokinetics, re-check levels at steady state (see above).
- Status epilepticus/parenteral administration: **Phenytoin:** 20 mg/kg, IV, at rate not exceeding 1 mg/kg/min, followed by maintenance of 100 mg 6–8 hourly.
  - Cardiac monitoring required due to risk of hypotension and cardiovascular collapse.
- **Fosphenytoin:** Prodrug of phenytoin, may be given IM.

Drugs and practical prescribing

Special requirements

- Formulation and dosing equivalence.
  - Phenytoin sodium and phenytoin base are not bioequivalent.
  - 100 mg phenytoin sodium (injection/capsules) ≈ 92 mg phenytoin base (suspension/infatab).
- Blood and skin disorders: Advise patients to look for signs of rash, fever, (AHS – see above) mouth ulcers, sore throat, bruising and bleeding (blood dyscrasias).

MICRO-monitoring

Phenytoin kinetics and plasma level monitoring toxicity

Therapeutic drug monitoring: see Ch. 2, Section 2.4.

- Therapeutic range: 10–20 mg/L.
  - Highly protein bound. Low total body protein levels may lead to toxicity within normal plasma range due to increased free drug.
- Levels timing: pre-dose (trough level).
- Initially follows first order kinetics. Zero order kinetics may occur within normal dose ranges, care required with dose changes. (See Ch. 1, and Ch. 2, Sections 2.2, 2.3, 2.4).
- Approximately 7–10 days to steady state.

TOPIRAMATE TOPAMAX®

- Likely Na^+ channel inhibition, GABA enhancement and antagonism of some sub-type glutamate receptors.
- Indicted for mono/adjuvant therapy for generalized tonic-clonic seizures and partial seizures with/without secondary generalization.

GABAPENTIN AND PREGABALIN

Pharmacodynamics

- GABA analogues but has no effect on the GABA system.
- Antiepileptic properties likely due to binding of the α_2-δ subunit of voltage-gated calcium channels in the central nervous system, reducing excitatory neurotransmitter release.
- Pregabalin may be associated with fewer side effects.

Indications

- Mono/adjuvant therapy of partial seizures with/without secondary generalization.
- Neuropathic pain.

Cautions

- Hepatic and renal disease.
- Abrupt withdrawal may lead to sweating, anxiety, nausea, pain.

Adverse effects

- Gastrointestinal: Diarrhoea, constipation, dyspepsia.
- Neurological: Dizziness, drowsiness, anxiety, cerebellar symptoms.
- Dermatological: Rash, Stevens-Johnson syndrome, hot flushes.
- Blood dyscrasias.

Important interactions

- Antiepileptic effect reduced by antidepressants and antipsychotics.

Examples

- **Gabapentin (Neurontin®)**
- **Pregabalin (Lyrica®)**

LAMOTRIGINE

Pharmacodynamics

- Likely Na⁺ channel inhibition and reduction in glutamate release.

Indications

- Mono/adjuvant therapy of partial seizures.
- Mono/adjuvant therapy of primary and secondarily generalized tonic-clonic seizures.
- Seizures associated with Lennox-Gastaut syndrome.

Cautions

- Hepatic and renal impairment, pregnancy, breast-feeding.
- Hypersensitivity reactions.

Adverse effects

- Hypersensitivity and dermatological: Rash or serious skin reaction may occur, DIC, multiorgan dysfuction (AHS) (see MICRO-facts above).
- Blood dyscrasias.
- Others: Cerebellar side effects, hepatic dysfunction, hallucinations.

Important interactions

- Antiepileptic effect reduced by antidepressants and antipsychotics.

Examples

- **Lamotrigine (Lamictal®)**

Special requirements

- Adverse effects: Counsel patients about rash (AHS/SJS) (see MICRO-facts above), bruising and bleeding (blood dyscrasias).

BARBITURATES AND RELATED DRUGS

- Phenobarbital (phenobarbitone) is the major barbiturate in clinical use.
- Primidone has some anticonvulsant action, but the effect is continued by its two major metabolites, one of which is phenobarbitone.
- Use is limited by sedative effects, tolerance and rebound seizures on withdrawal.
- Hypersensitivity reactions may also occur (see MICRO-facts above).
- Principle action is potentiation of GABA by binding to $GABA_A$ receptors.
- Indicated in all forms of epilepsy except absence seizures.
- Used in status epilepticus (see below).
- CYP450 enzyme induction can cause multiple drug interactions.
- Examples:
  - **Phenobarbital**
  - **Primidone**
  - **Thiopentone** (very short acting barbiturate used in anaesthesia)

BENZODIAZEPINES

- Clonazepam and clobazam are occasionally used in epilepsy as they are believed to be more effective at reducing seizures compared to their sedation profile.
- However, as tolerance occurs over weeks to months their effects often wane.

Pharmacodynamics, cautions, adverse effects

- See Section 8.5.

Examples and dosing

- **Clonazepam:**
  - All forms of epilepsy.
  - Also indicated in status epilepticus (see below) and myoclonus.
- **Clobazam:**
  - Adjunct in epilepsy.
  - Anxiety (short term), given at night.

MICRO-print

Other antiepileptics

- **Ethosuximide [Emeside®]**
  - Inhibits thalamic calcium channels (see mechanism of action above).
  - Commonly used for typical absence seizures and occasionally for atypical absences and myoclonic or tonic seizures.
- **Lacosamide (Vimpat®):** Licensed for adjuvant treatment of partial seizures with/without secondary generalization.
- **Levetiracetam (Keppra®):** Licensed for mono/adjuvant therapy for partial seizures with/without secondary generalization, and for adjunctive therapy of myoclonic seizures and primary generalized tonic-clonic seizures.
- **Rufinamide (Inovelon®):** Licensed for adjunctive treatment of Lennox-Gastaut syndrome.
- **Tiagabine (Gabitril®):** Adjunctive for partial seizures with/without secondary generalization.
- **Vigabatrin (Sabril®):** Restricted adjuvant for partial seizures with/without secondary generalization when other combinations not tolerated.
- **Zonisamide (Zonegram®):** Adjunctive for refractory partial seizures with/without secondary generalization.

STATUS EPILEPTICUS

First line treatment

- The regimen used will depend upon the setting:
  - IV access difficult e.g. in the community.
    - Buccal midazolam 10 mg (unlicensed) may be considered first line.
    - Rectal diazepam 10–20 mg as alternative.
  - IV access obtainable e.g. in hospital.
    - Lorazepam 4 mg IV as slow bolus over 2 minutes is considered first line and may be repeated once if necessary.
    - Diazepam 10 mg IV over 2 minutes can be used as a shorter acting alternative.
    - Preferably give the less irritant emulsion **Diazemuls®**.

Second line treatment

- **Phenytoin**, or the less irritant fosphenytoin may be used (see above).
- Alternatively, phenobarbitol sodium may be used.

Drugs and practical prescribing

Refractory epilepsy
- This may require intubation and anaesthetic agents.

Other agents
- **Paraldehyde** may still be used occasionally, particularly in children.
- The most common route is rectal, though it may be given IM.
- Respiratory depression is less pronounced compared to benzodiazepines.

8.4 ANTIPSYCHOTIC (NEUROLEPTIC) MEDICATIONS

GENERAL PRINCIPLES

Pathophysiology of schizophrenia and antipsychotic medications
- Psychotic symptoms of schizophrenia are likely due to excessive dopaminergic activity in the mesolimbic system.
- This excess may be:
  - Physiological i.e. schizophrenia.
  - Secondary to alterations of dopaminergic balance (e.g. L-dopa causing acute psychotic reactions).
- To date, five receptors within the CNS for dopamine have been identified, called D_{1-5}.
- For the majority of antipsychotic drugs the predominant clinical effect is thought to be due to antagonism of dopamine D_2 receptors.
- Interactions with 5-HT, α-adrenoceptors and other dopamine receptors also occur to varying degrees with the neuroleptics and affect efficacy and adverse event profile.

Classification of antipsychotics
First generation (typical) antipsychotics
- Broadly categorized as phenothiazine and non-phenothiazine (see below).
- High affinity for D_2 receptors is associated with good control for positive symptoms but less effective for negative symptoms.
- Generally have more sedative, extrapyramidal and more antimuscarinic effects than second generation 'atypical' drugs.
- Main uses:
  - Acute psychomotor agitation, particularly when sedation required.
  - Short-term control of agitation, where conservative methods failed.
  - Schizophrenia where tolerated and effective.
  - Non-psychiatric disorders (e.g. nausea in palliation, choreas/tics, intractable hiccups).

Second generation (atypical) antipsychotics

- Lower affinity for D_2 receptors.
  - Similar effect for positive symptoms compared to 'first generation drugs'.
  - Improved efficacy for negative symptoms.
- Reduced extrapyramidal effects compared to 'first generation drugs'.
- Differing activity at range of receptors other than D_2 gives each drug distinct clinical profiles (for both efficacy and adverse effects).
- Main uses:
  - Acute and chronic psychoses (acute – olanzapine, risperidone).
  - Short-term control of aggression (see individual drugs for licensing).
  - Mania (usually limited to acute setting).

Adverse effects

- Dopamine antagonism related.
  - 'Extrapyramidal' movement disorders are associated with dopamine antagonism within the basal ganglia.
    - Effects are dose dependent and increased in drugs with high receptor affinity.
      - Parkinsonism (including tremor).
      - Akasthisia (restlessness).
      - Tardive dyskinesia ('lip-smacking', may be irreversible).
      - Dystonia and dyskinesia.
    - Dystonias and parkinsonism may be treated with *antimuscarinics* (see Section 8.1).
- Endocrine hormone disturbances:
  - Hyperprolactinaemia secondary to reduced dopamine antagonism at the pituitary gland (less common with second-generation drugs).
  - Hyperglycaemia and diabetes.
- α-adrenoceptor blockade: Orthostatic hypotension.
- Antimuscarinic symptoms: See Section 8.1.
- Other notable side effects:
  - Neuroleptic malignant syndrome (see below).
  - Drowsiness, dizziness, cardiovascular symptoms (including hypotension, arrhythmias), ECG changes (pre-prescription ECG advised), blood dyscrasias, cholestatic jaundice, hypercholesterolaemia (with second generation drugs).

Drugs and practical prescribing

MICRO-facts

Neuroleptic malignant syndrome
- Rare but potentially life threatening condition thought to be due to reduction in dopamine levels or D_2 receptor blockade.
- It is more common with first generation antipsychotics, but may also result from use of the second generation 'atypicals'.
- It results in hyperthermia, muscle rigidity and autonomic instability (including tachycardia and unstable blood pressure).

Choice
- For both acute and chronic treatment, choice is largely based upon:
  - Patient response.
  - Prevalence of positive or negative symptoms.
  - Adverse effect profile: For sedative effect use first-generation drugs (e.g. chlorpromazine).
- Depot preparations of some drugs may ensure concordance and aid maintenance therapy. Those available include:
  - **Fluphenazine, haloperidol, flupentixol, zuclopenthixol, pipotiazine, haloperidol, risperidone, paliperidone, olanzapine.**
- Other than **clozapine**, all antipsychotics are generally considered to be of equivalent efficacy.
- Pre-prescription ECG, FBC, LFT ± cholesterol monitoring advised. Routine follow up monitoring is also good practice.

FIRST GENERATION 'TYPICAL' ANTIPSYCHOTICS

Pharmacodynamics
- See above.

Indications
- See above and individual drug profiles.

Contraindications
- CNS depression, coma, phaeochromocytoma.

Cautions
- Cardiovascular disease (tachycardia, hypotension and QT prolongation with some drugs).
- Parkinson's disease (antagonism of dopaminergic effects).
- Elderly (susceptible to side effects, use low doses. Also, risk of stroke in those with dementia).
- Hepatic/renal impairment, pregnancy, breast-feeding, risk of antimuscarinic effects (BPH, angle-closure glaucoma), myasthenia gravis, history of jaundice or blood dyscrasias, epilepsy/reduced seizure threshold.

Adverse effects
- See above.

Important interactions
- Anti-arrhythmics and tricyclic antidepressants: risk of QT prolongation/ arrhythmias.
- Antiepileptics: Reduction in seizure threshold.
- Potentiation of hypotensive and sedative effects of other drugs.

Examples
Phenothiazine derivatives
- **Chlorpromazine (Largactil®)**
  - Commonly used for its sedative effects.
  - Schizophrenia/psychoses (including acute – 25–50 mg, IM).
  - Other indications include anti-emetic in palliative care.
  - Risks of contact sensitization, workers should avoid direct contact with tablets.
- **Levomepromazine (Nozinan®)**
  - Similar to chlorpromazine.
  - Nausea in palliative care (common use).
  - May be administered orally or via s/c infusion.
- **Prochlorperazine**
  - Less sedating than chlorpromazine but with more extrapyramidal effects.
  - Nausea and vomiting (common use – oral, 20 mg stat, then 5–10 mg TDS).
    - **Stemetil®** oral, **Buccastem®** buccal (useful when oral route not tolerated).
  - Other indications include labyrinthine disorders, schizophrenia and psychoses.
- Other phenothiazine derivatives:
  - **Promazine, pericyazine, pipotiazine, fluphenazine, perphenazine, trifluoperazine.**

Butyrophenones
- Less sedation, hypotension and antimuscarinic effects than with chlorpromazine but more association with extrapyramidal events.
- Used for agitation and restlessness but only where conservative methods have failed.
- **Haloperidol (Haldol®, Serenace®)**
  - Schizophrenia and other psychoses: 0.5–3 mg 2–3 times daily.
  - Agitation/restlessness in elderly: 0.5–1.5 mg OD/BD, oral.

- Acute agitation/psychosis: 2–10 mg, 4–8 hourly, IV/IM (half dose in elderly), max 18 mg in 24 hours.
- Other indications: Severe anxiety, intractable hiccup, nausea in palliation.
- **Benperidol (Anquil®):** Control of deviant antisocial sexual behaviour.
- **Droperidol (Xomolix®):** Post-operative nausea and vomiting.

Thioxanthenes

- Less sedation but associated with extrapyramidal events.
- **Flupentixol:** Schizophrenia, oral and depot (**Depixol®**); depression: **Fluanxol®**.
- **Zuclopethixol:**
  - Schizophrenia/psychoses tablets and depot (**Clopixol®**).
  - As zuclopenthixol acetate (**Clopixo accuphase®**) IM, acute psychoses.

Substituted benzamides

- **Sulpiride (Dolmatil® Sulpor®).** High doses for positive symptoms. Low doses are effective for apathetic patients; however use with caution as aggravates agitation.

SECOND GENERATION 'ATYPICAL' ANTIPSYCHOTICS

Pharmacodynamics

- See above.
- Each individual drug's receptor binding characteristics affects clinical profile (see below).

Indications

- See above and individual drug profiles.

Contraindications and cautions

- As for first-generation antipsychotics.

Important interactions

- As for first-generation antipsychotics.

Adverse effects

- See above for general side effects.
- Less extrapyramidal effects compared with first generation drugs.
- Each individual drug's receptor binding characteristics affects the clinical profile (see below).

Examples

- **Amisulpride (Solinan®)**
  - Selective mesolimbic D_{2+3} antagonist.
  - Used in schizophrenia (including negative symptoms) and acute psychosis.

- **Olanzapine (Zyprexa®)**
  - Commonly used for schizophrenia, mania and agitation.
  - Limiting side effects include hyperglycaemia and diabetes.
- **Risperidone (Risperdal®)**
  - Licensed for psychosis, mania and persistent aggression in Alzheimer's disease.
  - Limiting side effects: Prolactin related (see above)
  - Also available as depot **Risperdal (Consta®)**
  - **Paliperidone (Xeplion®)** metabolite of risperidone, IM, licensed for maintenance of schizophrenia
- **Quetiapine (Seroquel®)** – XL m/r
  - Licensed in schizophrenia and bipolar disorder.
  - Antagonistic effects at various histamine, dopamine, serotonin and adrenergic receptors.
- **Aripiprazole (Abilify®)**
  - Partial agonist at D_2 receptors and lowers prolactin levels.
  - Licensed orally for schizophrenia, treatment and recurrence of mania. IM preparation available for control of disturbed behaviour/agitation in schizophrenia.
  - Side effect profile: little weight gain and no prolactin related effects compared to other drugs.
- **Clozapine (Clozaril®)**
  - $D_1 > D_2$ antagonism.
  - Effective in resistant psychosis.
  - Licensed in resistant schizophrenia and psychosis in Parkinson's disease.
  - Use limiting side effects (drug previously withdrawn):
    - Patient, prescriber and pharmacist must be registered with brand specific monitoring services before they are prescribed and dispensed.
    - Agranulocytosis: requires frequent monitoring and patient education.
    - Also myocarditis, cardiomyopathy and bowel pseudo-obstruction.

8.5 HYPNOTIC AND ANXIOLYTIC MEDICATIONS

GENERAL PRINCIPLES

- The drugs used as anxiolytics (for anxiety) and hypnotics (for sleep disturbance) are intrinsically related, and consequently have overlapping effects.
- Acute management of both usually involves a benzodiazepine or related drugs.
- As these often lead to tolerance (increased dose requirements) and dependence (addictive potential) their usefulness and appropriateness is limited in the chronic setting.

- Withdrawal effects include rebound phenomena (anxiety, insomnia) and seizures (usually after high doses).
- The sedative action of hypnotic drugs does not lead to physiological sleep, and withdrawal effects mimic the initial problem.
- Many of these drugs have multiple uses as anxiolytics, hypnotics, antiepileptics, muscle relaxants and adjuvants in alcohol withdrawal.
- Sedative actions are also used in cases of acute psychosis, aggression and agitation associated with a variety of psychiatric disorders.

BENZODIAZEPINES

Pharmacodynamics

- Enhance action of the neurotransmitter GABA by binding to $GABA_A$ ligand gated Cl^- channels.
- Increased intracellular Cl^- transfer leads to neuronal hyperpolarization and inhibition of action potentials.

Pharmacokinetics

- Distribution/elimination:
  - Elimination mainly renal.
  - Half-lives vary and alter clinical profile:
    - Drugs with short half-lives are used as hypnotics to avoid morning hangover effects. Withdrawal effects tend to be more pronounced.
    - Drugs with longer half-lives are used as anxiolytics. They lead to daytime somnolence and have higher potential to accumulate in hepatic/renal impairment.

Indications

- See below for patterns of individual drug use.
- Short term (2–4 weeks) as anxiolytics and hypnotics.
- Panic attacks.
- Alcohol withdrawal.
- Seizures.
- Muscle relaxants.
- Sedation ± amnesiac properties (pre-operative or procedural sedation).
  - Amnesic properties drug dependant – see profiles below.
- Acute drug induced dystonia.

Contraindications

- Respiratory depression.

Cautions

- Respiratory disease: Muscle weakness and myasthenia gravis.
- Hepatic and renal dysfunction: Consider dose reduction, risk of accumulation.

- History of drug or alcohol abuse.
- Elderly (susceptible to side effects – start at half normal dose).
- Driving: Sedative effects may affect performance of skilled tasks.

Adverse effects

- Hangover effects: Drowsiness and lightheadedness (warn patient of driving risk).
- Neurological: Sedation, confusion, ataxia, coordination disturbance (particularly in elderly).
- Others: Dependence, withdrawal, risk of respiratory depression (at high doses).
- Muscle weakness.

Important interactions

- Enhanced hypotensive and sedative effects of other drugs.

Examples

Anxiolytics

- **Diazepam:** Long acting benzodiazepine (see pharmacokinetics above).
  - Anxiety: 2 mg TDS initially, oral; with insomnia 5 mg ON.
    - PR, IM, IV (see below) also available.
  - Muscle relaxant: Dose as per anxiety.
  - Acute anxiety/panic attacks/alcohol withdrawal.
  - Other indications: Seizures (see Section 8.3), febrile convulsions, adjunct in alcohol withdrawal, pre/perioperative use.
  - IV: risk of thrombophlebitis, reduced using emulsion formulation **Diazemuls®**.
- **Chlordiazepoxide:** Long acting benzodiazepine (as per diazepam)
  - Anxiety.
  - Alcohol withdrawal (common use).

MICRO-facts

Chlordiazepoxide reducing regimens
- Use local policies: usually start at 10–20 mg QDS + PRN and transition down smoothly over around 7 days.
- Be willing to review the patient's requirements and adjust the dose up or down as needed.
  - Reducing regimens are not a 'one size fits all' prescription.
- For example: 20 mg QDS then 20 mg TDS, 15 mg TDS, 10 mg TDS, 5 mg QDS, 5 mg BD, 5 mg OD.
- Max daily dose normally 200 mg.
- Caution in those with hepatic impairment, consider lorazepam in this group instead.

Drugs and practical prescribing

- **Lorazepam:** Short-acting benzodiazepine preferred in hepatic/renal impairment.
  - (Acute use only due to profound withdrawal and dependence).
    - Anxiety: 1–4 mg daily in divided doses, oral.
    - Acute anxiety/panic attacks.
    - Other indications: pre/perioperative, seizures (see Section 8.3); alcohol withdrawal in hepatic disease (unlicensed).
- Other anxiolytics: **Alprazolam, Oxazepam.**

Hypnotics

- **Temazepam:** Short-acting benzodiazepine (see pharmacokinetics above), 10–20 mg ON, oral (max 40 mg).
- **Nitrazepam:** Prolonged action compared to tempazepam – risk of hangover effects.
- Other hypnotics: **Flurazepam** (prolonged action), **loprazolam** and **lormetazepam** (short action).

MICRO-print

Benzodiazepine overdose

- **Flumazenil** is a very short-acting antagonist at the benzodiazepine receptor.
- It may be used to reverse the effects of benzodiazepines but only under close supervision.
- Caution is required as most benzodiazepine overdoses can be managed conservatively, and flumazenil may cause seizures, flushing and anxiety.

Other benzodiazepines

- **Midazolam:**
  - Water soluble benzodiazepine.
  - When given IV, high peak concentrations are associated with anterograde amnesia. Useful for sedation with amnesia during some procedures.
  - Other uses: Status epilepticus, anaesthesia, sedation in intensive care/anaesthesia.
- **Clonazepam, Clobazam**: Epilepsy (see Section 8.3).

NON-BENZODIAZEPINE HYPNOTICS (Z-DRUGS)

- The Z-drugs are short acting, non-benzodiazepine medications which bind to the benzodiazepine receptor on the $GABA_A$ Cl$^-$ channels.
- Claimed reduced propensity for tolerance.
- **Zopiclone (Zimovane®)** 3.75–7.5 mg ON, oral; may lead to taste disturbance.
- Others: **Zaleplon** (very short acting), **zolpidem**.

> **MICRO-reference**
> National Institute for Health and Clinical Excellence. *Insomnia - newer hypnotic drugs: review decision.* Technology appraisals TA 77. London, UK: NICE, 2004. Available from: http://www.nice.org.uk/TA077

> **MICRO-print**
> **Other anxiolytics**
> - **Buspirone:**
>   - Thought to act as a partial agonist at $5HT_{1A}$ receptors.
>   - Licensed for short-term management of anxiety with or without depression.
>   - Low dependence potential.
> - **Meprobamate:** Not used due to low efficacy, hazard in overdose and dependence.
> - Antidepressants: Some tricyclic antidepressants and SSRIs may be used in long-term anxiety where benzodiazepines would lead to tolerance and dependence. The MAOI moclobemide is indicated in social anxiety disorder (see Section 8.2).
> - β-blockers: Some use for reducing autonomic symptoms of anxiety.

> **MICRO-print**
> **Other hypnotics**
> - **Clomethiazole (Hemineverin®):** Short acting, reduces hangover effects and it is therefore appropriate in the elderly. Also used in alcohol withdrawal in the in-patient setting, and may be given IV in status epilepticus.
> - Antihistamines: Sedative antihistamines may be of some use. **Promethazine (Phenergan®)** is sold over the counter and is sometimes used in children.
> - **Chloral hydrate:** Now used in a very limited role.
> - **Sodium oxybate:** Licensed for narcolepsy with cataplexy (under specialist supervision).
> - **Melatonin:** A pineal hormone which may aid sleep patterns. Licensed in the UK for short-term therapy for insomnia in adults over the age of 55.
> - Barbiturates: **Amobarbital** and **butobarbital** are only indicated for intractable insomnia in those already taking barbiturates. They have some role in epilepsy (see Section 8.3).

Drugs and practical prescribing

8.6 MEDICATIONS FOR BIPOLAR DISORDER AND MANIA

GENERAL PRINCIPLES

Bipolar affective disorder

- The presence of mania, with or without the presence of depressive episodes.
- Antidepressants should be used with caution during the depressive episode as they may induce mania.
- Treatment options are aimed at:
  - Acute mania control.
  - Prophylaxis of mania and bipolar disorder.

Acute mania control

- Involves use of a mood stabilizer (lithium/valproate – see below) in combination with antipsychotics for marked behavioural disturbance.
- Antipsychotics may be required as the mood stabilizers take time to elicit their effects.
- **Olanzapine**, **quetiapine** or **risperidone** (see Section 8.4) are common first line medications. **Asenapine** is a second-generation antipsychotic also licensed in bipolar disorder.
- **Lithium** or **valproate** are used either as augmentation to antipsychotics if needed, or continued as a patients' normal medication. Effective lithium levels should be confirmed (see below).
- Acute behavioral disturbances or agitation may be treated with a benzodiazepine such as **lorazepam** (see Section 8.5).

Prophylaxis of mania and bipolar disorder

- **Lithium** or **valproate** are considered first line therapies for acute mania and prophylaxis of bipolar disorder.
- **Valproate** is licensed for this use as the semi-sodium salt **Depakote**®. Sodium valproate may be used, but is unlicensed (see Section 8.3).
- **Carbamazepine** may be used for rapid cycling bipolar disorder under specialist supervision (see Section 8.3).

MICRO-reference
National Institute for Health and Clinical Excellence. *The management of bipolar disorder in adults, children and adolescents, in primary and secondary care.* Clinical guideline CG38. London, UK: NICE, 2006. Available from: www.nice.org.uk/CG38

LITHIUM

Pharmacodynamics

- Precise mechanism unknown.
- Likely to involve cellular second-messengers.

Pharmacokinetics

- Requires serum-lithium concentration monitoring (see below).
- Elimination:
    - Excreted via the kidneys in the urine by the same mechanism as sodium.
    - Low sodium concentrations in the renal tubules allow increased reuptake of lithium and potentially toxic levels.
    - Elimination half-life 12–24 hours, varies with formulation therefore prescribe as brand.

Indications

- Prophylaxis and treatment of mania.
- Prophylaxis of bipolar disorder.
- Recurrent depression (specialist use only).

Cautions

- Conditions of sodium imbalance (see pharmacokinetics).
- Cardiac disease and QT prolongation.
- Others: Pregnancy and breast feeding, elderly (reduce dose), myasthenia gravis, abrupt withdrawal.

Adverse effects

- General:
    - Fine tremor.
    - Hypothyroidism.
    - Gastro-intestinal disturbance.
    - Symptoms of nephrogenic diabetes insipidus (polyuria, polydipsia).
    - Others: Weight gain, hyperparathyroidism, hypokalaemia, leucocytosis, ECG changes.
- Toxicity related:
    - Mild: Severe fine tremor, diarrhoea, nausea, reduced concentration.
    - Moderate: Vomiting, ataxia, slurred speech, coarse tremor, disorientation.
    - Severe: Seizures, confusion, coma, circulatory collapse.

Important interactions

- Drugs which affect sodium balance or renal function (e.g. diuretics, ACE inhibitors, NSAIDs).
- Amiodarone (note thyroid effects and ECG changes).

Examples

- **Lithium carbonate: Camcolit®, Liskonium®, Priadel®**
- **Lithium citrate: Li-Liquid®, Priadel**

Special requirements

- Serum-lithium concentration, renal and thyroid function should be monitored prior to initiation and then every 6–12 months once stable.

MICRO-monitoring

Lithium monitoring and toxicity

- Therapeutic drug monitoring: See Ch. 2, Section 2.4.
  - Therapeutic range: 0.4–0.8 mmol/L (up to 1.0 in acute mania).
  - Levels timing: Pre-dose (trough level).
    - Weekly until stable, then 3 monthly.
  - Follows first order kinetics.
  - Approximately 5–7 days to steady state.
  - Toxicity: mild 1.0–1.5 mmol/L, moderate 1.5–2.0 mmol/L, severe >2.0 mmol/L.
- See adverse effects above.

8.7 CNS STIMULANTS

GENERAL PRINCIPLES

- CNS stimulants are most commonly used in the treatment of narcolepsy and attention deficit hyperactivity disorder (ADHD).
- In ADHD they should be initiated under specialist advice and act as psychostimulants, thought to increase alertness and attentiveness.
- Precise mechanisms vary with individual drugs and are discussed below.
- They act as indirect sympathomimetics increasing synaptic cleft levels of neurotransmitters (noradrenaline and/or dopamine) via indirect mechanisms.
- This increase in amine levels is responsible for their therapeutic as well as adverse effects.

Examples and dosing

- **Atomoxetine (Strattera®)**
  - Inhibits noradrenaline re-uptake into presynaptic terminals.
  - Licensed for ADHD.
  - Risk of hepatic disorders, suicidal ideation and QT prolongation.

- **Dexamphetamine (Dexedrine®)**
  - Increases noradrenaline and dopamine levels in synaptic cleft.
  - Likely mechanism is reuptake inhibition and increased release via displacement of neurotransmitters from storage in presynaptic terminal.
  - Licensed for refractory ADHD and narcolepsy.
- **Methylphenidate (Ritalin®), MR – Concerta XL®, Equasym XL®, Medikinet XL®**
  - Thought to block reuptake of dopamine and noradrenaline.
  - Licensed in ADHD, used unlicensed for narcolepsy.
- **Modafinil (Provigil®)**
  - Pharmacodynamics unknown, likely to increase monoamine levels.
  - Licensed for excessive sleepiness in narcolepsy with or without cataplexy.

8.8 DRUG USE IN DEMENTIA

GENERAL PRINCIPLES

- These drugs decrease the rate of cognitive decline in Alzheimer's disease and should normally be prescribed by specialists.
- Effects should be assessed by 3-monthly cognitive assessments to ensure their use is appropriate for both effect and severity of dementia.
- There are currently two main classes of drugs:

Acetylcholinesterase inhibitors

- These drugs decrease synaptic acetylcholine degradation thereby enhancing neurotransmission.
- Three drugs are available:
  - **Donepezil (Aricept®)** and **galantamine (Reminyl®):** Licensed for mild to moderate dementia in Alzheimer's disease.
  - **Rivastigmine (Exelon®):** Licensed for mild to moderate dementia in Alzheimer's and Parkinson's disease.

MICRO-print

Acetylcholinesterase selectivity

- The above drugs are more selective for central acetylcholinesterases than those in the peripheral nervous system.
- This distinguishes them from those more selective for the neuromuscular junction nicotinic acetylcholinesterases which are used in myasthenia gravis and anaesthesia.

NMDA receptor antagonist

- Current theories suggest excessive glutamate levels in Alzheimer's disease may lead to neuronal death via excitotoxicity.
- Antagonism of glutamate's receptor (NMDA) by **memantine (Ebixa®)** may be beneficial in moderate to severe dementia.

Antipsychotics

- Second generation, 'atypical' antipsychotics may be used to control aggression and psychosis in Alzheimer's disease.
- This use, however, is associated with increased mortality and stroke (see Section 8.4).

8.9 DRUG USE IN SUBSTANCE DEPENDENCE

Alcohol dependence

- **Disulfram (Antabuse®)** is used as an adjunct in alcohol dependence. It blocks the metabolism of acetaldehyde (a metabolite of alcohol) by inhibiting acetaldehyde dehydrogenase. When alcohol is consumed with the drug, the increased levels of acetaldehyde cause flushing, vomiting, palpitations and hypotension.
- **Acamprosate (Campral®)** unknown mechanism of action. Used in maintenance of alcohol dependence.
- The benzodiazepines **chlordiazepoxide** and, **lorazepam** and **clomethiazole** are used to reduce withdrawal symptoms (see Section 8.5).

Smoking cessation

- Nicotine replacement therapy is considered the first line in combatting smoking.
- **Bupropion (Zyban®)** has been used as an antidepressant and may be used for those targeting a 'quit date'.
- **Varenicline (Champix®)** is a selective nicotine receptor partial agonist.

Opioid dependence

- Should be managed under a multi-disciplinary team with specialist care.
- **Methadone:** See Ch. 10, Section 10.4.
- **Buprenorphine:** See Ch. 10, Section 10.4.
- **Naltrexone** is an opioid antagonist given to former addicts to prevent relapse.
- **Lofexidine (BritLofex®)** provides symptomatic relief due to reduction in sympathetic tone. Similar to clonidine but with less hypotension (see Ch. 5, Section 5.5).

Drugs and practical prescribing

9 Endocrinology

9.1 TREATMENT OF DIABETES

GENERAL PRINCIPLES

- Diabetes mellitus is a condition associated with insufficient action of insulin. It is divided into two major categories:
  - Type 1 – A total lack of insulin production likely due to autoimmune destruction of β-cells within the islets of Langerhans of the pancreas.
    - Treatment will always require insulin therapy.
  - Type 2 – A relative lack of insulin production combined with cellular resistance to its action.
    - Treatment options after dietary and lifestyle control may:
      - Enhance insulin production.
      - Reduce systemic insulin resistance.
    - Ultimately insulin therapy may be required, and due to resistance insulin requirements may be significantly higher than in type 1 disease.

> **MICRO-references**
> National Institute for Health and Clinical Excellence. *Type 2 diabetes: the management of type 2 diabetes (update)*. Clinical Guidance 66. London, UK: NICE, 2008. Available from: http://guidance.nice.org.uk/CG66
>
> National Institute for Health and Clinical Excellence. *Type 2 diabetes – newer agents (a partial update of CG66): short guideline*. Clinical Guidance 87. London, UK: NICE, 2011. Available from: http://guidance.nice.org.uk/CG87

INSULIN

- See Chapter 16.

ANTI-DIABETIC MEDICATIONS

Biguanides (metformin)

- Requires residual β-cell function as it does not stimulate insulin release. It therefore rarely causes hypoglycaemia.
- Commonly used as it also aids weight reduction.

Pharmacodynamics

- Reduces hepatic glucose production by inhibiting gluconeogenesis and glycogenolysis.
- Increases insulin sensitivity, improving peripheral glucose uptake and utilization.
- Delays intestinal glucose absorption.

Indications

- Type 2 diabetes mellitus (ideally following dietary/lifestyle changes). Polycystic ovary syndrome (unlicensed): associated with metabolic syndrome and insulin resistance.

Contraindications

- Ketoacidosis.
- Lactic acidosis (see below).

Cautions

- Renal impairment (requires monitoring, see lactic acidosis below).

Adverse effects

- Gastrointestinal: Common – anorexia, nausea, vomiting, diarrhoea (usually transient)
- Others: Abdominal pain, taste disturbance, lactic acidosis (see below).
- Rarely: Hepatitis, pruritus, urticaria, reduced vitamin B absorption.

Examples

- Start at low doses and increase slowly to avoid the common gastrointestinal effects.
- **Metformin (Glucophage®)** 500 mg–2 g daily in divided doses (BD-TDS), oral.
- **Metformin MR, Glucophage SR®** dose as above in 1–2 divided doses.
    - Reduced GI side effects due to peak concentrations.
    - Bioavailability approximately equivalent allowing 1:1 dose conversion.
- Combination preparations: with **pioglitazone: Competact®**, with **sitagliptin: Janumet®**, with **vildagliptin: Eucreas®**.

Special requirements
- Renal impairment:
  - **Metformin** use in renal impairment may lead to lactic acidosis, a rare but serious side effect.
  - Reduce dose with eGFR <45 mL/min/1.73m^2 and avoid with eGFR <30 mL/min/1.73m^2.
  - Treatment should be stopped in the presence of acute kidney injury.
  - Metformin should be stopped prophylactically:
    - On the day of surgery.
    - Prior to use of iodine containing contrast media (e.g. for CT/MRI) due to risk of contrast induced nephropathy. May restart after 48 hours if U+E are at baseline levels.

Sulphonylureas
- Class of drugs commonly used in type 2 diabetics who:
  - Are not overweight (induces weight gain, in contrast to metformin).
  - Have particularly high glucose levels.
- Augment insulin secretion and may cause hypoglycaemia.
  - Usually associated with excessive dose or in the elderly.
  - More common with long acting sulphonylureas (see below).

Pharmacodynamics
- Stimulation of insulin secretion by functioning pancreatic β-cells, with significant post prandial action.
- Action at their receptor blocks the ATP-dependent K$^+$ channels of β-cells.
- The resulting depolarization initiates Ca^{2+} influx and insulin secretion.

Indications
- Type 2 diabetes mellitus.
- Commonly used second line with/without metformin dependant on glucose control.

Cautions and contraindications
- Elderly: Risk of hypoglycaemia.
- Hepatic and renal impairment: Risk of hypoglycaemia, risk of cholestatic jaundice.
- Others: Ketoacidosis.

Adverse effects
- Gastrointestinal (mild/infrequent): Nausea, vomiting, diarrhoea and constipation.
- Others: Hypoglycaemia, hepatic dysfunction, initial hypersensitivity reactions.

Drugs and practical prescribing

Examples

- **Gliclazide:** Short acting, half-life 6–14 hours
  - 40–80 mg OD/BD, oral (max 320 mg daily)
  - Note: **Diamicron MR®** clinical effect 30 mg MR = 80 mg normal release
- **Tolbutamide:** Short acting, half-life 4–8 hours; considered safer in elderly
- Others: **Glipizide (Minodiab®)** and **glimepiride (Amaryl®)** are short acting, **chlorpropramide** and **glibenclamide** are long acting and not recommended.

OTHER ANTI-DIABETIC MEDICATIONS

Acarbose

- Used when there is lack of tolerance of other agents or for post-prandial hyperglycaemia.
- Leads to dose-dependent reduction of carbohydrate metabolism through competitive inhibition of intestinal enzymes (α-glucosidases).
- Gastrointestinal side effects including flatulence are limiting factors.
- **Acarbose (Glucobay®).**

Thiazolidinediones (glitazones)

- **Pioglitazone** may be used in combination with metformin, sulphonylureas or insulin under the guidance of an experienced physician.
- Associated with increased incidence of heart failure and bladder cancer.
- Associations with heart failure lead to the suspension of **rosiglitazone**.

Pharmacodynamics

- Reduces insulin resistance, likely due to interactions with specific nuclear receptors within liver, fat and skeletal muscle cells leading to increased sensitivity.

Indications

- Type 2 diabetes mellitus as monotherapy or in combination with metformin/sulphonylureas.

Contraindications

- History of heart failure or bladder cancer (including uninvestigated macroscopic haematuria).

Cautions

- Cardiovascular disease: Risk of heart failure.
- Hepatic impairment: Risk of liver dysfunction – requires monitoring.
- Others: Pregnancy and breast-feeding, increased risk of bone fractures.

Adverse effects

- General: Weight gain (common), oedema, anaemia, headache, visual disturbance.

- Others: Hypoglycaemia, fatigue, insomnia, vertigo, sweating, altered blood lipids, proteinuria, bladder cancer, liver toxicity (see above).

Examples

- **Pioglitazone (Actos®)**
- With **metformin, Competact®**

Special requirements

- Monitor liver function, cardiovascular and bladder cancer risk as above.

Meglitinides (Glinides)

- Rapid onset and short acting, orally administered drugs which should be taken shortly before meals.

Pharmacodynamics

- Stimulate insulin release in the same mechanism as sulphonylureas but with a distinct binding site (see sulphonylureas above).

Indications

- See examples.

Cautions and contraindications

- Ketoacidosis.
- During intercurrent illness and surgery substitute these drugs for insulin.
- Elderly/malnourished patients.

Adverse effects

- Hypoglycaemia.
- Hypersensitivity reactions.

Examples

- **Nateglinide (Starlix®)** licensed in type 2 diabetes mellitus in combination with metformin only. Available as tablets.
- **Repaglidine (Prandin®)** licensed for type 2 diabetes mellitus as monotherapy or in combination with metformin. Available as tablets.

Dipeptidylpeptidase (DPP-4) inhibitors (gliptins)

- These are second-line medications (see MICRO-reference earlier in chapter).

Pharmacodynamics

- DPP-4 is an enzyme which degrades the incretins GLP-1 (glucagon like peptide-1) and GIP (glucose-dependent insulinotropic polypeptide).
- Inhibition of DPP-4 increases incretin levels with two hypoglycaemic effects:
  - Enhanced β-cell sensitivity to glucose by both enzymes, increasing insulin production.

* Enhanced α-cell sensitivity to glucose by GLP-1 increasing glucose-appropriate glucagon secretion.

Indications

* Type 2 diabetes mellitus.
  * As monotherapy or in combinations with metformin, sulphonylureas, pioglitazone or insulin.
* Specific licensing varies with individual drugs.

Contraindications

* Ketoacidosis.

Cautions

* See individual drug profiles.

Adverse effects

* General: Gastrointestinal disturbance, peripheral oedema, headache, tremor asthenia.
* Less common/rare: Constipation, arthralgia, hypoglycaemia, upper respiratory tract infection, nasopharyngitis, pancreatitis.
* See individual drugs for further adverse effects.

Examples, specific cautions and special requirements

* **Sitagliptin (Januvia®)**:
  * May cause cutaneous vasculitis, Stevens-Johnson syndrome.
  * Discontinue if symptoms of acute pancreatitis.
* **Vildagliptin (Galvus®)**; with metformin **Eucreas®**
  * Caution in hepatic dysfunction (monitor liver function) and heart failure (avoid if moderate or severe).
* Others: **Linagliptin (Trajenta®), saxagliptin (Onglyza®)**.

GLP-1 (glucagon like peptide-1) receptor agonists

* These are second line medications administered by subcutaneous injection.
* For advice on use see MICRO-reference earlier in chapter.

Pharmacodynamics

* GLP-1 receptor agonists which increase insulin secretion, suppress glucagon secretion, and slow gastric emptying.
* Mechanism of action is similar to the DPP-4 inhibitors.

Indications

* Type 2 diabetes mellitus in combination with other therapies.

Contraindications

* Ketoacidosis, inflammatory bowel disease, diabetic gastroparesis.

Cautions
- Elderly, pancreatitis, renal impairment (may require cessation of therapy), hepatic impairment (avoid with liraglutide only).

Adverse effects
- General: Gastrointestinal disturbance, weight loss, hypoglycaemia, gastro-oesophageal reflux disease headache, asthenia, injection-site reactions.
- Less common/rare: Pancreatitis (may be severe, inform patients of symptoms).

Examples, specific cautions and special requirements
- **Exenatide (Byetta®):** S/C administration
  - MR preparation also available as **Bydureon®**, weekly administration.
- **Liraglutide (Victoza®):** S/C administration

Special requirements
- Counsel patients to seek medical attention if symptoms of pancreatitis develop.

9.2 TREATMENT OF THYROID DISORDERS

THYROID HORMONES

- The thyroid hormones thyroxine (T_4) and tri-iodothyronine (T_3) are produced and released by the thyroid gland in response to stimulation by the anterior-pituitary hormone, thyrotrophin stimulating hormone (TSH).
- TSH release is in turn stimulated by hypothalamic production of thyrotrophin-releasing hormone (TRH).
- Systemic circulation of T_3 and T_4 exerts a negative feedback effect at both the hypothalamus and the pituitary.
- Most circulating thyroid hormone exists bound to plasma proteins, but only the free hormone proportion is responsible for their physiological effects.
- In medical use T_4 is the mainstay of thyroid hormone replacement therapy with its extended action. T_3 has a shorter half-life and is used when a rapid action is required.

Pharmacodynamics
- T_4 is considered a prohormone of T_3, with T_3 being the active hormone.
- Free T_3 and T_4 enter cells upon which most T_4 is converted into T_3.
- T_3 binds and activates specific nuclear receptors affecting gene transcription and protein synthesis leading to increased cellular metabolism.

Pharmacokinetics
- Distribution/elimination: T_4 has a long half-life (around 7 days) facilitating daily administration.

- T_3 has a shorter elimination half-life due to reduced protein binding compared to T_4. This leads to a more a rapid effect seen within hours of administration.

Indications

- Thyroid replacement therapy in hypothyroidism (myxoedema).
- Diffuse non-toxic goitre.
- Others: Hashimoto's thyroiditis, thyroid carcinoma, neonatal hypothyroidism.

Contraindications

- Thyrotoxicosis.

Cautions

- Elderly (risk of occult cardiac disease).
- Cardiovascular disorders (risk of precipitating angina/arrhythmias).
- Long-standing hypothyroidism.
- Diabetes insipidus.
- Also see special requirements.

Adverse effects

- Adverse effects are related to physiological function and usually indicate excessive dosage.
  - Cardiac: Arrhythmias, palpitations, tachycardia, angina.
  - GI: Diarrhoea, vomiting.
  - Others: Flushing, sweating, weight loss, restlessness.

Examples

- **Levothyroxine** (thyroxine sodium). Tablets and oral solution available.
  - Doses are started with around 1.6 μg/kg (lower in elderly/cardiovascular disease – see above).
  - Dose is titrated to symptoms and TSH levels (aiming normal limits). Repeat tests are required approximately 1 month after dose changes and at routine follow-up.
- **Liothyronine** (L-tri-iodothyronine sodium), available oral. IV preparation used for hypothyroid coma.

Special requirements

- Baseline ECG required due to risk of cardiovascular complications.
- Diabetes mellitus: Increased anti-diabetic requirements.
- Panhypopituitarism: Initiate corticosteroid therapy prior to levothyroxine.

THIONAMIDES (ANTI-THYROID THERAPY)

- These drugs render hyperthyroid patients euthyroid when used at high dose over a period of 4–8 weeks.

- Carbimazole is used first line. Propylthiouracil has a higher incidence of agranulocytosis, and is used in patients with sensitivity to carbimazole.

Pharmacodynamics

- **Carbimazole** is a prodrug which is converted into the active compound methimazole.
- **Propylthiouracil** is the active moiety itself.
    - In addition to the common mechanism below it also reduces peripheral conversion of T_4 to T_3.
- These active thionamide moieties competitively inhibit thyroid peroxidase.
    - This enzyme oxidizes iodide, allowing incorporation of iodine into the precursor of the thyroid hormones, thyroglobulin.

Indications

- Maintenance therapy for hyperthyroidism.
    - Continued for around 18 months before thyroid state is assessed without medication.
    - High dose to render euthyroid then titrated down to maintenance dose.
    - As a 'block and replace regimen':
        - High doses are used in combination with replacement thyroid hormone therapy.
        - Reduces the risk of hypothyroidism associated with titrated maintenance dosing.
- Pre-thryroidectomy treatment to reduce the risk of peri-operative thyrotoxicosis due to thyroid hormone release.
    - β-blockers are also used to counteract peripheral effects.
- Treatment of thyrotoxic crisis (see below).

Cautions and contraindications

- Carbimazole: contraindicated in severe blood disorders.
- Hepatic and renal impairment.

Adverse effects

- Mild GI disturbance including nausea.
- Taste disturbance.
- Malaise.
- Headache.
- Hepatitis.
- Blood dyscrasis (see MICRO-facts below).

Examples

- See above.

Drugs and practical prescribing

> ### MICRO-facts
>
> **Neutropenia and agranulocytosis with thionamide therapy**
> Patients should report signs of bone marrow suppression or infection (including sore throat). If suspected a full blood count should be requested, and treatment stopped if neutropenia is discovered.

> **MICRO-print**
> **Iodine and iodide**
> - These compounds reduce the vascularity of the thyroid gland through mechanisms not well understood.
> - They may be used:
>   - Pre-operatively in combination with a thionamide.
>   - In thyrotoxic crisis (see below).
> - They are not used in maintenance therapy as the anti-thyroid effect diminishes with time.
> - Radioactive iodine (I^{131}) is used in the treatment of thyrotoxicosis.
> - Aqueous iodine oral solution (*Lugol's iodine*): Iodine 5%, potassium iodide 10%.
>
> **Thyrotoxic crisis ('thyroid storm')**
> - This condition may arise following surgery, radioactive iodine therapy or in infection.
> - Leads to hyperpyrexia, tachycardia/arrhythmias, vomiting and diarrhoea.
> - This may lead to dehydration, coma and death.
> - Treatments aim to reduce thyroid hormone production, and protect from their peripheral effects.
> - This involves IV fluids, cooling, glucocorticoids, Lugol's iodine, β-blockade, thionamides and treatment of arrhythmias.

9.3 CORTICOSTEROID THERAPY

GENERAL PRINCIPLES

- In humans, corticosteroids are endogenous hormones produced by the adrenal cortex.
- They are divided into two main categories:
- Mineralocorticoids:
  - Principally aldosterone, produced in the zona glomerulosa.

- Act upon the intra-nuclear steroid receptors of the distal tubules and collecting ducts of nephrons resulting in:
  - Na$^+$ (and consequently water) retention.
  - H$^+$ and K$^+$ secretion into the urine.
- Glucocorticoids:
  - Principally cortisol, produced in the zona fasciculata.
  - Through intracellular mechanisms they act at nuclear receptors, affecting gene transcription.
  - The main actions are:
    - Anti-inflammatory/immunosuppression:
      - Inhibition of pro-inflammatory mediators including prostaglandins and leucotrienes via suppression of phospholipase A2 and COX-2 production.
      - Repression of macrophage and lymphocyte function.
      - Reduction of IL-2 levels and interactions with leukocyte cell surface receptors preventing activation and extravasation into tissues.
    - Carbohydrate metabolism.
  - Glucose levels are raised by:
    - Insulin antagonism (peripheral resistance).
    - Glycogenolysis.
    - Gluconeogenesis: Direct stimulation of the liver, and promotion of the precursors via catabolism of protein (muscle, skin) and fat
      - Other:
        - Cortisol has significant mineralocorticoid-like effects.
- With regard to therapeutics, other additional actions are mainly associated with adverse effects and are discussed below.

MICRO-facts

Glucocorticoid equivalences
These doses are for equivalent glucocorticoid action and do not reflect any mineralocorticoid activity:

- Short acting: Hyrdocortisone 20 mg.
- Intermediate acting: Methylprednisolone 4 mg, prednisolone 5 mg, triamcinolone 4 mg.
- Long acting: Betamethasone 750 micrograms, dexamethasone 750 micrograms.

Adapted from: Joint Formulary Committee. *British National Formulary.* 66th ed. London: BMJ Group and Pharmaceutical Press; 2014.

Drugs and practical prescribing

GLUCOCORTICOIDS

- Glucocorticoids are used therapeutically for their anti-inflammatory and immunosuppressive actions or in adrenal replacement.
- Each of the synthetic steroids varies with regard to their degree of anti-inflammatory and mineralocorticoid activity.
- Systemic corticosteroid preparations are discussed here; see below regarding locally active preparations.

MICRO-print

Local effects of corticosteroids

- In order to reduce the adverse effects and complications associated with systemic corticosteroids, local administration should be chosen if at all possible.
- For this reason corticosteroids are available in a variety of locally acting formulations.
- This includes:
    - Various creams, ointments, buccal mucosal, opthalmological and ENT preparations.
    - Inhalers in respiratory conditions (see Ch. 6, Section 6.3).
    - Enemas and locally acting oral preparations in IBD (see Ch. 7, Section 7.2).
    - Intra-articular injections for rheumatological and orthopoedic conditions.

Pharmacodynamics

- Intra-nuclear effects on gene transcription.
- Due to this intra-nuclear mechanism anti-inflammatory effects are not seen for 6-8 hours after administration.

Indications

- Specific indications are discussed under individual drug profiles.
- Adrenal replacement therapy.
- Anti-inflammatory/immunosuppressive actions used either locally or systemically for a wide variety of conditions.

Cautions and contraindications

- Adrenal suppression and withdrawal: see below.
- Infections:
    - Increased susceptibility and severity with prolonged courses.
    - Particular care with sepsis, tuberculosis (TB) (including reactivation of dormancy), chickenpox, measles and live vaccines.

> **MICRO-print**
> **Other cautions with corticosteriod therapy:**
> - Psychiatric reactions: Particularly in patients with a history of mental health disorders (see adverse effects below).
> - Others: Children (growth restriction), osteoporosis, hypertension, recent MI (risk of myocardial rupture), diabetes mellitus, CCF, glaucoma, ocular infections, epilepsy, peptic ulcer, hypothyroidism, history of steroid myopathy, ulcerative colitis, diverticulitis, recent intestinal anastomoses, VTE, myasthenia gravis

Adverse effects

Adverse effect profile varies with the relative gluco-/mineralo-corticoid activity of the drug.

- Gastrointestinal: Dyspepsia, oesophageal ulceration, acute pancreatitis, candidiasis.
- Musculoskeletal: Proximal myopathy, osteoporosis, tendon rupture, avascular necrosis.
- Endocrine: Hyperglycaemia, menstrual irregularities, hirsuitism, weight gain (polyphagia).
- Psychiatric: Insomnia, euphoria, irritability, mood lability, psychosis, suicidal thoughts.
- Ophthalmic: Glaucoma, papilloedema, cataracts, corneal thinning, exacerbation of infections.
- Steroid specific: Cushing's syndrome (at doses above physiological levels).
- Others: Leucocytosis, VTE; also see cautions above.
- Mineralocorticoid: Features of Conn's syndrome (hypertension, Na^+ and water retention, hypokalaemia, hypocalcaemia and H^+ loss).

Examples

- **Hydrocortisone:**
    - Glucocorticoid with significant mineralocorticoid activity.
    - Uses:
        - Acute management of asthma and IBD, hypersensitivity reactions.
            - 100–500 mg TDS-QDS, IV.
            - Note oral prednisolone 5 mg ≡ hydrocortisone 20 mg IV.
        - Replacement therapy (often with fludrocortisone).
        - Intra-articular injections for rheumatological conditions.
        - Topical as low potency steroid for dermatological, opthalmological and otological conditions and haemorrhoids.
- **Prednisolone:**
    - Predominately exerts a glucocorticoid effect.

- Four times more potent than hydrocortisone.
- Oral formulations only.
- Uses:
  - Suppression of inflammatory and allergic disorders in acute and maintenance therapy.
  - Immunosuppressant.
  - Palliation (enhance appetite and sense of well-being).
  - Anti-tumour effect in some haematological cancers.

- **Dexamethasone:**
  - Extremely potent glucocorticoid with negligible mineralocorticoid effects.
  - Oral and injectable forms available.
  - Uses:
    - Suppression of inflammatory and allergic disorders.
    - Diagnosis of Cushing's disease (dexamethasone suppression test).
    - Cerebral oedema associated with malignancy.
    - Also used in pulmonary and cerebral oedema with altitude sickness.
    - Nausea and vomiting with anaesthetics, chemotherapy and palliation.
    - Congenital adrenal hyperplasia.
    - Also used to prevent respiratory distress syndrome in premature babies by prenatal administration to mother.
    - Adjuvant in bacterial meningitis.

- **Betamethasone:** Similar to dexamethasone as betamethasone sodium phosphate, as betamethasone esters (e.g. valerate) it has marked topical effects.
- **Methylpredisolone:** Methylated variant of prednisolone available as parenteral formulations.
- **Deflazocort:** Derived from prednisolone with a high glucocorticoid activity.
- **Triamcinolone:** Used as an IM depot injection an in various topical formulations.

Special requirements

- Advice to patients:
  - Adrenal suppression and withdrawal risks (see below).
  - Immunosuppression (infection risk including severe chickenpox and measles – avoid contact and seek medical attention if exposure).
  - Mood and behaviour changes.
- Other serious effects as detailed above.

MICRO-facts

Adrenal suppression and withdrawal of glucocorticoids

- Prolonged therapy leads to adrenal suppression and atrophy.
- This may lead to adrenal insufficiency, hypotension and death in two settings:
  - **Diminished adrenocortical response:** Additional steroids must be administered during intercurrent illness, trauma or surgical procedures. 25–50 mg IV is often administered, and continued TDS for 24–72 hours if significant adrenal compromise is expected (e.g. moderate/major surgery).
  - **Withdrawal:** In those unlikely to relapse, dose reduction may be rapid to a physiological level (≈ 7.5 mg prednisolone), then withdrawn slowly to avoid adrenal insufficiency.
    - Indications for this include repeated courses, courses >3 weeks, dose >40 mg prednisolone, repeated doses in the evening.

MINERALOCORTICOIDS

- **Fludrocortisone (Florinef®):**
  - Corticosteroid with high mineralocorticoid activity mimicking endogenous aldosterone.
  - Its therapeutic and adverse effects are similar to other corticosteroids, but with marked mineralocorticoid and diminished glucocorticoid activity.
  - It is around 500 times more potent a mineralocorticoid than hydrocortisone.

Indications

- Mineralocorticoid replacement therapy in adrenal insufficiency (Addison's disease).
- Postural hypotension: Na+ retaining activity (unlicensed indication).

10 Analgesia

10.1 PRINCIPLES OF PRESCRIBING ANALGESIA

- Pain is a common issue that can be difficult to assess due to its subjective nature.
- In prescribing analgesia you must consider the pain's source (cause) and course (time line).

CAUSES OF PAIN

- The pathophysiology of pain is centred on the 'pain gateway'.
- Peripheral inputs from nociceptors (pain receptors) and tactile receptors interact with suppressive inputs from descending pathways from the brain (higher control).
- Via interactions with the modulating substantia gelatinosa inter-neurones within the dorsal horn, the overall summative pain stimulus is transmitted to higher centres via the spinothalamic tract.
- It is through these pathways which both pain and analgesics have their effect.
- Pain itself is usually initiated in two ways:
    - Simulation of the various types of nociceptors (nociceptive pain).
    - Direct neuronal stimulation or irritation (neuropathic pain).

STRATEGIES FOR PAIN SUPPRESSION

- To remove pain you may either suppress it (analgesia) or inhibit sensory pathways (anaesthesia).
- This may be achieved using the following approaches.

Nociception

- Decrease nociceptive input:
    - Reduce inflammatory chemicals (e.g. NSAIDs).
    - Reduced nociceptive input (e.g. capsaicin).
    - Modulation – tactile input competes with nociceptive input via the substantia gelatinosa reducing spinothalamic excitation. For example:
        - Rubbing the site of injury reduces pain.
        - TENs machines.

> **MICRO-print**
> **Reduction in nociceptive input and capsaicin**
> **Capsaicin** initially opens heat-sensitive calcium channels leading to sensation of heat, but with prolonged stimulation depletes levels of the noxious neurotransmitter Substance P.

Block primary afferent

- Local anaesthetics block voltage-gated Na^+ channels, stopping the action potential and conduction of pain signals.

Interact with high level perception

- Interference with perception of pain via modulation of higher functions within the brain, or interactions with the descending pathways.
- For example, opioids, ketamine, some anticonvulsants and antidepressants.

TIME LINE OF PAIN

- The temporal nature of pain (i.e. acute or chronic) is an important consideration that will influence the prescription of pain relief.

Chronic pain

- Effective strategies for managing chronic pain will depend upon the cause.
- In most cases the World Health Organisation (WHO) pain ladder provides a good starting approach. Originally designed for cancer pain, the rules may be extrapolated to a wide variety of conditions (Fig. 10.1).

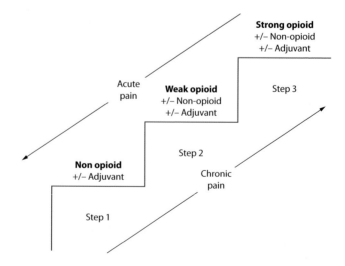

Fig. 10.1 WHO pain ladder.

- In chronic pain, analgesia should be started at step 1 (unless patient presents with acute exacerbation – see below).
- Start with simple non-opioid analgesia and add other appropriate medication as required.
  - Simple analgesia includes paracetamol, nefopam and NSAIDs.
  - Weak/moderate opioids include codeine, dihydrocodeine and tramadol.
  - Strong opioids include morphine, oxycodone and fentanyl.
- These medications can be supplemented with agents not typically associated with pain relief, known as 'adjuvant analgesia'.
- Adjuvants may be introduced at any level of the ladder and should be tailored to the pathogenesis of the pain:
  - Inflammatory conditions: NSAIDs.
  - Dull, visceral pain: Opioids.
  - Neuropathic pain: Anti-epileptics (e.g. gabapentin).
  - Bone pain:
    - Responds better to NSAIDs than opioids.
    - In neoplastic bone metastases, bisphosphonates and radiotherapy may also be effective.
  - Compressional pain (e.g. due to oedema surrounding tumours): May respond well to steroids such as dexamethasone.

Rational prescribing of analgesia

- Choice:
  - Treatment should be guided by analgesic effect and patient tolerance of the medication.
  - All analgesic medications are associated with different adverse effect profiles that some patients may not be able to tolerate.
  - It is common for patients to have to switch opioids due to adverse effects.
- Breakthrough pain:
  - If this is occurring regularly then consider an increase in the regular dose.
  - PRN analgesia should always be prescribed with regular analgesia.
  - Patients may require higher doses of PRN medication as their regular dose increases.
  - A good approach is to use a sixth of the regular dose up to six times daily.
    - For example, if a patient takes morphine sulphate M/R 60 mg BD (total daily dose 120 mg), a reasonable PRN dose is 20 mg, up to 6 doses daily.
- Weak opioids:
  - Unlike strong opioids these have a 'ceiling effect' of analgesia.

Drugs and practical prescribing

- Pains uncontrolled on one weak opioid will unlikely benefit from addition of another.
  - Never prescribe two weak/moderate opioids together for pain as this will simply increase side effects without additional analgesia.
- If one is not effective at maximum dose consider a strong opioid, or addition of appropriate adjuvants.

Acute pain

- Acute pain should be treated according to the severity, however it is still appropriate to use the WHO pain ladder as a guide.
- In contrast to chronic pain, acute pain typically works 'down the ladder', providing adequate initial pain relief and subsequently titrating the dose downwards.
- For short-term management of acute pain, strong or fast acting analgesia may be considered.
- Consider opioids, or in obstetrics/painful procedures an inhaled nitrous oxide/oxygen (50/50) mix ('gas and air').

Post-operative pain

- A special case of acute pain which may be difficult to manage.
- If severe pain is expected patient controlled analgesia (PCA) may be prescribed.
- This involves the use of a syringe driver (usually containing an opioid) to deliver an IV bolus when the patient presses a button.
  - Maximum rates of delivery apply via lockout periods to prevent overdose, and background infusions may be considered for those inadequately controlled with boluses.
- Anaesthetists often use epidurals or administer analgesics during surgery to ensure good initial post-operative analgesia.
- These frequently run as a background infusion with/without patient controlled bolus facility PCEA (patient controlled epidural analgesia).

10.2 SIMPLE ANALGESIA

DRUG PROFILES

Paracetamol

Pharmacodynamics

- Analgesic effect believed to be due to centrally interfering with descending serotonergic pain pathways, possibly mediated either by COX inhibition or via cannabinoid receptors.
- Reduction in prostaglandin synthesis may account for the antipyretic effect.

Indications

- Mild pain, or in conjunction with other analgesics in more severe pain.
- Antipyretic.

Cautions and contraindications
- Hypersensitivity to paracetamol or any of its constituents.
- Hepatic dysfunction.

Adverse effects
- Very rare in normal doses.
  - Blood dyscrasias.
  - Hypersensitivity.
  - Hepatic dysfunction – in overdose (see below).

Important interactions
- Occasionally significant enhancement of coumarin's (warfarin) effect.

Dosing
- Patients over 12 years:
  - Patients >50 kg: 0.5–1 g 4–6 hourly to max 4 g daily, PO/IV/PR.
  - Patients <50 kg: 15 mg/kg 4–6 hourly.

Special requirements
- Reduce dose to max 3 g daily in patients with chronic alcoholism, hepato-cellular deficiency, chronic malnutrition or dehydration.
- Consider similar dose reduction in frail elderly.
- Renal excretion delayed if eGFR <30 mL/min.
- Infusion dose: Minimum dose interval 6 hours as opposed to 4 hourly for oral.

MICRO-facts

Paracetamol overdose (OD)

- If taken as a single dose, significant hepatotoxicity may occur in those who have taken more than 150 mg/kg.
- However, overdose may occur at lower doses, particularly in the elderly and those with other risk factors (as above), or if other substances have been taken.
- In staggered overdose any paracetamol level simply confirms ingestion. If there is any concern regarding potential toxicity then treatment should be initiated as below.
- In overdose normal conjugation pathways of metabolism in the liver become saturated.
  - This leads to increased levels of the toxic metabolite NABQI which is produced via the alternative CYP450 metabolic pathway.
  - NABQI is initially mopped up by the antioxidant glutathione. When stores of this are depleted the metabolite causes hepatotoxicity and renal tubular necrosis.

continued...

> *continued...*
>
> - Treatment
>   - Activated charcoal if overdose taken within 1 hour.
>   - Replete glutathione stores with IV N-acetylcysteine or oral methionine.
>   - Most effective if given less than 8 hours following OD.
>   - Some benefit up to 24 hours.
>   - Treat as per dosage schedule (see BNF/Toxbase/local protocols).
>   - Note levels not accurate in staggered overdose.
> - If there is any doubt, treatment should be initiated.

Nefopam

Pharmacodynamics

- Mechanism of action not well understood, but is distinct from other analgesics.
- Thought to be centrally acting, inhibiting re-uptake of neurotransmitters potentiating the descending pathways.

Indications

- Mild to moderate pain.
  - May be used in conjunction with other analgesics.
  - Does not cause respiratory depression if opiates are of concern.
- Not indicated in MI as increases myocardial oxygen demand.

Cautions and contraindications

- Patients with epilepsy (decreases seizure threshold).
- Patients taking MAOIs (increases amine levels leading to a risk of hypertension and psychosis).

Adverse effects

- Anticholinergic effects (common): Dry mouth, blurred vision, urinary retention, tachycardia.
- Others: Hallucinations, insomnia, nausea, harmless pink discolouration of the urine.

Important interactions

- Monoamine oxidase inhibitors.

Dosing

- 60 mg TDS, oral (30 mg elderly); range 30–90 mg TDS.

Special requirements

- Elderly particularly susceptible to central side effects (hallucination/confusion).

10.3 NON-STEROIDAL ANTI-INFLAMMATORY DRUGS (NSAIDs)

- Analgesics frequently used for their antipyretic and anti-inflammatory actions.
- Aspirin also used as an antiplatelet drug (see Ch. 5, Section 5.7).

DRUG PROFILES

Pharmacodynamics

- NSAIDs inhibit the enzyme cyclo-oxygenase (COX).
- COX converts arachadonic acid into prostaglandin H2 (PGH2), which via further enzymatic transformation is converted into the functional end products:
  - Prostaglandins (PG): Mainly PGE2 and PGI2 (aka prostacyclin) whose functions include:
    - Sensitizing nociceptors to bradykinin thereby exacerbating sensation of pain.
    - Producing gastric mucus and bicarbonate secretion.
    - Vasodilation at the afferent arteriole of the glomerulus regulating glomerular filtration pressure.
    - Natriuretic effect (hence inhibition leads to salt and water retention).
    - Prostacyclin also decreases platelet aggregation.
  - Thromboxane A_2
    - Released by activated platelets.
    - Leads to vasoconstriction and increased platelet aggregation.
- Inhibiting these factors gives NSAIDs both their therapeutic and adverse effects; described below.
- NSAIDs reversibly inhibit COX through hydrogen bonds, with the exception of aspirin which irreversibly binds via acetylation.
- COX exists in two isoforms.
  - COX-1:
    - A constitutive enzyme present in many tissues.
    - COX-1 inhibition is responsible for the adverse effects (and antiplatelet effect) of NSAIDs.
  - COX-2:
    - Induced in tissues subjected to inflammation.
    - COX-2 inhibition results in anti-inflammatory actions.
- Differential selectivity for COX-1 or 2 governs NSAIDs side effect profile.

> **MICRO-print**
>
> **NSAIDs and COX selectivity versus specificity**
>
> - NSAIDs side effect profile is related to their individual affinities for COX-1 or COX-2.
> - No drug is specific for either enzyme.
> - Greater selectivity of a drug for COX-2 confers lower GI and renal side effects and higher anti-inflammatory effect, due to COX-2 inducement in areas of inflammation.
> - Unfortunately, COX-2 selective inhibitors have shown increased incidence of myocardial infarction and strokes with many now withdrawn from the market.

Indications

- Pain relief, particularly acute and chronic inflammation.
    - Headaches, dysmenorrhoea, bone pain and musculoskeletal pains respond well to NSAIDs.
    - Full anti-inflammatory effect may not be seen for up to 3 weeks.
- Treatment of acute gout
    - Naproxen and diclofenac commonly used.
    - Ibuprofen has insufficient anti-inflammatory action.
    - Aspirin contraindicated due to increased uric acid retention in kidney.

Cautions and contraindications

- Severe heart failure (due to risk of fluid retention).
- Asthmatics due to risk of bronchospasm (see below).
- Elderly, dehydration, concomitant ACEi – see Fig. 10.2.
- Risk of thrombotic events (MI and stroke).
    - Particularly COX-2 inhibitors, diclofenac (150 mg daily) and high dose ibuprofen (2400 mg daily).
- Selective COX-2 inhibitors contraindicated in IHD.
- All NSAIDs contraindicated in active PUD, non-selective NSAIDs contraindicated in previous PUD.
- Tiaprofenic acid is cautioned in urinary tract disorders due to risk of cystitis.

Adverse effects

- Gastrointestinal discomfort: Nausea and diarrhoea.
- Gastrointestinal bleeding: Systemic (PG related) and local effect related (see MICRO-facts).
    - Local effects may be partially relieved by enteric coating or administration with food/milk.
- Hypersensitivity:
    - Rashes, angioedema, bronchospasm.

* Bronchospasm in asthmatics due to increased production of leucotrienes as alternative pathway for arachadonic acid conversion due to decreased PG production by NSAIDs. Not all asthmatics are sensitive to NSAIDs.
* Renal impairment: Through vasoregulatory mechanism or direct renal toxicity (see MICRO-facts).
* Fluid retention: May exacerbate heart failure.

MICRO-facts

NSAIDs and gastro-protection

* Reduce risks:
    * Use lowest dose for shortest time.
    * Consider alternatives.
* Prescribe gastro-protection if there is increased risk of adverse GI effects, for example:
    * Using the maximum recommended dose of an NSAID.
    * Age over 65 years.
    * History of gastroduodenal ulcer, GI bleeding, or gastro-duodenal perforation.
    * Concomitant use of medications that are known to increase the likelihood of upper GI adverse events (e.g. anticoagulants, aspirin [even low-dose], corticosteroids, and antidepressants (SSRIs, venlafaxine, or duloxetine).
    * Serious comorbidity, such as cardiovascular disease, hepatic or renal impairment (including dehydration), diabetes, or hypertension.
    * Prolonged NSAID use (e.g. OA, RA, chronic low back pain in those >45 years).
* Additional risk factors for NSAID-induced GI adverse events include:
    * The type of NSAID used.
        - Risk lowest with ibuprofen, intermediate with diclofenac, naproxen, indomethacin, ketoprofen, piroxicam and high with azapropazone.
    * The presence of *Helicobacter pylori* infection.
    * Excessive alcohol use.
    * Heavy smoking.
* PPIs should be used for gastro-protection (e.g. lansoprazole 15–30 mg daily or omeprazole 20 mg daily).

More information at: National Institute for Health and Clinical Excellence. *NSAIDs, prescribing issues*. Clinical Knowledge Summaries. London, UK: NICE CKS, 2013. Available from: http://cks.nice.org.uk/nsaids-prescribing-issues#!scenariorecommendation:3. (accessed 30/03/2014)

Important interactions

- NSAIDs may reduce excretion of methotrexate.
- Diuretics:
  - Increased risk of nephrotoxicity.
  - Hyperkalaemia with spironolactone and potassium-sparing diuretics.
- Reduced excretion of lithium.

Examples and dosing

- **Ibuprofen:** 200–400 mg 3–4 times daily initially, oral max 2.4 g daily.
- **Indomethacin:** 50–200 mg daily in divided doses, oral (PR 100 mg once to twice daily).
- **Diclofenac sodium:** Associated with higher cardiovascular risk (see COX-2s).
  - **Diclofenac potassium:** Rapid action.
- Others: **Piroxicam** (experienced physicians only due to serious GI and skin reactions), **ketoprofen, mefanamic acid, meloxicam, naproxen.**
- COX-2 selective inhibitors: **Celecoxib:** 100–200 mg in 1–2 divided doses, max 200 mg BD, oral.
  - Others: **Acemetacin, dexketoprofen, etodolac, etoricoxib, fenoprofen, flurbiprofen, nabumetone, sulindac, tenoxicam, tiaprofenic acid.**
- **Parecoxib** and **ketorolac:** Injectable forms for post-operative use.

MICRO-facts

NSAIDs and renal impairment

- NSAIDs may cause direct toxicity to the kidney i.e. interstitial nephritis.
- Reduced vasoconstriction at the glomerular afferent arteriole also leads to risk of acute renal failure secondary to hypoperfusion (see Fig. 10.2).
- Those at high risk include the elderly, dehydrated (including diuretic use) and those on ACEi (reduced efferent arteriolar vasoconstriction leads to inability to maintain perfusion pressures).

continued...

continued...

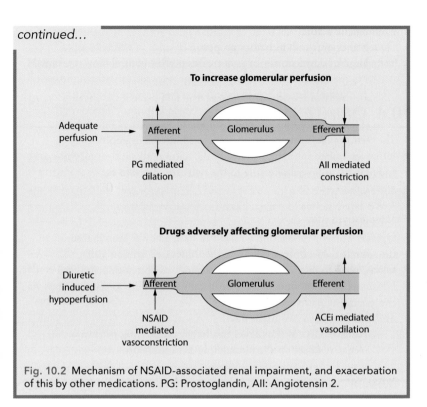

Fig. 10.2 Mechanism of NSAID-associated renal impairment, and exacerbation of this by other medications. PG: Prostoglandin, AII: Angiotensin 2.

CHOICE OF NSAID

- **Ibuprofen:**
    - Frequently used as a first choice NSAID.
    - Decreased side effects compared to other NSAIDs but also decreased anti-inflammatory action.
    - **Ketoprofen** similar but with increased side effects, dexibuprofen is the active enantiomer.
- **Naproxen:**
    - Good efficacy and decreased side effects compared to other NSAIDs but greater than ibuprofen.
    - NSAIDs with similar action include:
        - **Diclofenac** (less favoured as risk of cardiovascular events, high COX-2 activity), **tiaprofenic acid, aceclofenac, etodolac, nambumetone, sulindac, tenoxicam** and **piroxicam.**
- **Indometacin:**
    - More effective agent.
    - Increased side effects compared with naproxen.

- **Mefanamic acid:**
    - Minor anti-inflammatory properties.
    - Used in dysmenorrhoea as decreases uterine contractions, presumably PG mediated.

10.4 OPIATES

- The terms opiate and opioid are often used interchangeably.
- However, opiate specifically refers to the natural alkaloids (morphine and codeine), with opioid referring to the synthetic derivatives.

DRUG PROFILES

Pharmacodynamics

- Opiates work by interaction within the 'pain gateway' based around the substantia gelatinosa (SG) inter-neurones (see Section 10.1).
- Opiate receptor agonism, via G-protein actions decreases neural cell activity.
- Ultimately they modulate the pain stimulus travelling to the thalamus via the ascending pathway.
- This is achieved in two main ways:
    - Positive effect at the higher inhibitory descending pathways.
    - Negative effect on the modulating SG interneurons.

MICRO-print

Opiate receptors

- Opioid receptors are found throughout the nervous system and other organs including the GI tract.
- Activation produces:
    - Positive effects in the higher centers.
    - Inhibitory effects at the pain gateway and intestinal tract (reducing motility).
- There are three main types, each responsible for different actions.
    - These are activated by endogenous mediators, including the endorphins, dynorphins and andencephalins.
- Receptor types:
    - μ: Most important for analgesic effect. Three subtypes exist:
        - μ1: Analgesia, dependence.
        - μ2: Respiratory depression, euphoria, reduced GI motility.
        - μ3: Actions unknown.
    - κ: Analgesia, dysphoria, sedation.
- δ: Analgesia, dependence, antidepressant.

Pharmacokinetics

- Metabolism: Hepatic, many undergo significant first-pass metabolism.
- Elimination: Via urine and bile.

Indications

- Pain: Effective for visceral pain, less effective for sharp/neuropathic pain.
- Cough suppression.
- Respiratory distress during end of life.
- Anti-motility (anti-diarrhoeals).
- Management of substance abuse.

Contraindications

- Class specific:
  - Acute respiratory depression.
  - Risk of paralytic ileus.
  - Raised intracranial pressure/head injury (interferes with pupillary assessment).
  - Comatose patients.
- Specific:
  - Pethidine contraindicated with MAOIs due to hyperpyrexia and unstable blood pressure.

Cautions

- Impaired respiratory function.
- Hypotension (including shock).
- Smooth muscle spasm causing urethral stenosis, biliary disease and prostatic hypertrophy.
  - Uncommon as primary cause, therefore often used in patients with these conditions.
- Inflammatory/obstructive bowel disease (risk of constipation).
- Myaesthenia gravis.
- Elderly, hepatic and renal impairment (reduce dose).
- Driving: Due to drowsiness and enhanced effects of alcohol.

Adverse effects

- Nausea and vomiting (worse in initial stages).
- Constipation.
- Large dose effects: Muscle rigidity, hypotension, respiratory depression (may require specific monitoring, particularly if high risk of potentiating brady/apnoea e.g. post operatively, and in the neonate).
- Others: Brady/tachycardia, euphoria/dysphoria, hallucinations, confusion, urinary retention, miosis, visual disturbance, histaminergic reactions, smooth muscle spasm.

Important interactions

- MAOIs: Avoid concomitant use, CNS effects and hyper/hypotension, particular care with pethidine.

Examples and dosing

Weak opioids

- **Codeine:**
  - Low affinity for opioid receptors.
  - Around 10% metabolized to morphine (variation in metabolism of codeine may significantly alter therapeutic and adverse effects).
  - Mild to moderate pain: 30–60 mg 4 hourly, max 240 mg daily, oral/IM.
  - Constipation is a limiting side effect.
- **Dihydrocodeine:**
  - Similar efficacy to codeine.
  - High doses associated with more nausea and vomiting.
- **Meptazinol:** Uncommonly used; claimed decreased risk of respiratory depression.
- **Tramadol:**
  - Weak opioid receptor agonist.
  - Centrally actions include inhibiting neuronal reuptake of noradrenaline and probably increasing serotonin release.
    - These actions potentiate the descending pathways of pain gateway.
  - Reduced respiratory depression, constipation and abuse potential.
  - Psychiatric reactions (including psychosis), seizures and hypotension limit use.
  - 50–100 mg 4–6 hourly, max 400 mg daily, oral/IV/IM.

Strong opioids

- **Morphine:**
  - Nausea and vomiting are common due to chemoreceptor trigger zone stimulation.
  - Increased smooth muscle tone may lead to biliary/sphincter of Oddi spasm, urine retention and constipation (in combination with reduced peristalsis).
  - Histaminergic effects: Pruritus, vasodilation (bronchoconstriction in asthma).
  - Hepatic glucuronidation yields active metabolites which accumulate in renal impairment.
  - SC: 10 mg (5 mg in elderly) 4 hourly; IV: 5 mg (reduced in elderly) 4 hourly.
    - May be administered more frequently if required.

- Oral: 5–10 mg 4 hourly initially (reduced in elderly).
  - Formulations: Oral morphine sulphate: solution **Oramorph**®
    10 mg/5 mL, or morphine sulphate tablets **Sevredol**®.
    - Note concentrated Oramorph 100 mg/5 mL preparation
      exists.
  - For chronic pain work out daily requirements from 24 hour usage,
    convert to oral dosing if applicable and then change to a MR
    preparation e.g. **Zomorph**® capsules, **MST Continus**®.
- **Diamorphine:**
  - More potent analgesic with more rapid effect compared to
    morphine.
  - Associated with less nausea and hypotension.
  - 5 mg (up to 10 mg in well-muscled patients) 4 hourly, IM/SC;
    half dose for slow IV administration.
    - Used in acute pain, post MI and also epidurally.
- **Buprenorphine:**
  - Partial agonist of µ receptors
  - Effective analgesic but antagonizes full agonists
  - Difficult to reverse with naloxone due to strong receptor binding
  - Increasingly used for the management of substance abuse
  - Well absorbed following sublingual administration
  - Pain:
    - IV/IM: **Temgesic**®
    - Patches:
      - **BuTrans**® 7-day patch (72 hours for clinical effect)
      - **Transtec**® 96 hours (24 hours for effect)
  - Substance abuse: **Subutex**®, with **naloxone: Suboxone**®
- **Oxycodone:**
  - Similar efficacy and side effect profile to morphine, may be better
    tolerated
  - 5 mg 4–6 hourly initially OD, oral **OxyNorm**® capsules and liquid
    5mg/5mL
    - MR preparation **OxyContin**® for BD administration
  - 1–10 mg 4 hourly, IV; 5 mg initially 4 hourly, SC
- **Pethidine:**
  - Prompt but short lasting analgesia
  - Infrequently used due to toxicity associated with accumulation
  - Less meiosis than morphine due to anti-muscarinic actions
  - Used in obstetrics as it doesn't reduce uterine activity
- **Fentanyl, Alfentanil, Remifentanil:**
  - Rapid acting derivatives of pethidine used during anaesthesia, and for
    acute pain in certain settings (including PCA use)

- Fentanyl and the more rapid acting alfentanil are short acting due to rapid distribution. High dose/long term use saturates the compartments prolonging effect.
- Remifentanyl is metabolized by tissue esterases resulting in a short half-life independent of dose or duration.
- Fentanyl:
  - IV for anaesthetic use, and in acute pain by trained personnel
  - Regular analgesia: **DurogesicDTrans®** patches:
  - Replace 72 hourly, around 24 hours for full clinical effect (see MICRO-print box below).
  - Breakthrough analgesia:
  - Tablets, lozenges and nasal spray available
- Alfentanil, Remifentanil: Licensed for anaesthetic/intensive care

---

MICRO-print

Transdermal patches

- Transdermal patches allow absorption of drug through the skin and into the systemic circulation, and are frequently used to provide effective analgesia for many patients.
- Absorption characteristics may be altered by factors such as skin temperature and effective patch contact.
- Importantly, time to onset, rate of drug release (and hence duration of action of the patches) may be altered by skin temperature.
- There are reports of significant opioid overdose in patients with fever, and this should be considered for patients at risk of this.

- **Methadone:**
  - Long duration of action allowing once daily administration
  - Less sedating than morphine
  - Additional NMDA antagonist properties may alleviate neuropathic pain
  - Opiate withdrawal: Dosed by specialists
  - Multiple reactions increasing risk of QT prolongation and arrhythmias
- Others: **Papaveretum, Dipipanone, Pentazocine, Tapentadol, hydromorphone**

Special requirements

- Tolerance and dependence
  - Tolerance results from repeated administration of opioid drugs.
    - Mechanism unclear, may involve desensitization and down-regulation of receptors.
    - Tolerant patients require higher doses for effect.

- Dependence occurs on abrupt withdrawal of opioids where endogenous opioids do not meet the receptors demands.
  - Sweating, restlessness, abdominal pain, diarrhoea and tachycardia are common.
  - In those with analgesic requirements, there is reduced likelihood of dependence and concerns regarding this should not stop opioids being prescribed.
- For patients who use opioids for management of addiction, prescribing analgesia should follow normal pathways.
  - It is considered that their normal daily dose should meet there daily demands, and additional analgesia should be prescribed on top of this as for any other patient with similar analgesic requirement.

OPIATE DOSE CONVERSION GUIDE

- Doses are based upon 24 hours of morphine and its equivalents.
  - **Morphine:**
    - Oral morphine 20 mg ≈ SC/IV morphine 10 mg; 2:1 ratio
  - **Diamorphine:**
    - Oral morphine 30 mg ≈ 10 mg diamorphine SC; 3:1 ratio
  - **Codeine/dihydrocodeine:**
    - Oral codeine/dihydrocodeine 240 mg ≈ oral morphine 20 mg; 12:1 ratio, i.e. 60 mg QDS codeine ≈ 10 mg BD morphine MR
  - **Oxycodone:**
    - Oral oxycodone 1–520 mg ≈ oral morphine 30 mg; ~2:1 ratio
    - SC/IV oxycodone 15 mg ≈ oral morphine 30 mg; Using 2:1 for cautionary approach
  - **Tramadol:**
    - Tramadol 400 mg daily ≈ 40 mg morphine; 10:1 ratio, no exact conversion is available
  - **Fentanyl:**
    - 25 micrograms/hour fentanyl patch ≈ 60 mg oral morphine; Conversion calculated for 24 hours of morphine
- When converting opioids use caution and prescribe a lower dose with additional PRN medication.
- Some manufacturer's recommendations may vary slightly.

MICRO-reference
Robert Twycross R, Wilcock A. *Palliative Care Formulary (PCF),* 4th edition. Nottingham: Palliativedrugs.com: 2011.

MICRO-facts

NSAIDs and renal impairment

- Opiate overdose
- Respiratory depression is the most important complication of opiate overdose.
- Treatment involves administration of an opiate antagonist such as **naloxone**.
- Prescribe 200–400 micrograms IV and titrate to response repeating at 2–3 minute intervals to a maximum of 10 mg.
- May give continuous infusion (initial rate 60% of resuscitative dose/hour). Dose approximately 5–10 micrograms/kg/hr.
- An alternative is **naltrexone** which is shorter acting.
- Be aware, naloxone is shorter acting than most of the opiates. Patients must be monitored to ensure they don't return to a state of clinical overdose.

11 Antimicrobials I: Antibacterials

11.1 PRINCIPLES OF ANTIBIOTIC THERAPY

STARTING ANTIBIOTIC THERAPY

Several factors should be considered before treatment with antimicrobial therapy is initiated:

- Is there clinical evidence of infection?
    - Features of SIRS/sepsis (see MICRO-facts).
    - Symptoms/signs of anatomical infection (for example pneumonia or cellulitis).
    - Are inflammatory markers raised?

MICRO-facts

SIRS and sepsis

SIRS (systemic inflammatory response syndrome) is a systemic inflammatory response mediated by cytokines. If this is seen in the presence of infection it is classified as *sepsis*.

The typical criteria are:

- Temperature: <36°C or >38°C.
- Tachycardia: >90 beats per minute.
- Tachypnoea: >20 breaths per minute (or $PaCO_2 < 4.3$ kPa).
- White blood cells: $<4 \times 10^9$ or $>12 \times 10^9$.

Sepsis can be further categorized:

- Severe sepsis: Sepsis with end organ dysfunction (e.g. raised lactate, oliguria).
- Septic shock: Severe sepsis with hypotension refractory to IV fluids.

- What microbiological samples should be taken?
    - Appropriate samples should ideally be taken before starting antibiotics to maximize the chance of identifying a causative organism.
    - Exceptions to this rule occur where obtaining samples may lead to an unacceptable delay in the initiation of antibiotic therapy (e.g. lumbar puncture for cerebrospinal fluid in bacterial meningitis).

- Is empirical antibiotic therapy required?
  - If antibacterial therapy cannot wait for a microbiological diagnosis then empirical broad spectrum antibiotic treatment is required to cover the likely causative organisms.
  - Empirical antibiotics should subsequently be adjusted based on microbiological diagnosis:
    - A narrow spectrum agent should be used where possible to minimize development of resistance and the potential for adverse effects.
    - Sensitivity testing allows selection of an effective agent.
- What duration of therapy is required?
  - The duration of treatment should be decided and documented before starting antibiotic therapy, taking into consideration the desired response to therapy.
  - This should subsequently be reviewed in light of clinical response.
  - Five days is sufficient for most infections.
    - Deep-seated infections or those where it is difficult to ensure adequate antibacterial delivery (e.g. bacterial endocarditis) will require more prolonged therapy.
- Is adjuvant treatment required?
  - Some infections require adjuvant therapy for adequate treatment:
    - Surgery: Usually debridement of non-viable tissue (necrotizing fasciitis, abscesses) or removal of infected prostheses.
    - Line removal: In bacteraemia associated with indwelling catheters.

SENSITIVITY AND RESISTANCE

Sensitivity testing and antibacterial activity

- For infections where an organism has been identified, sensitivity testing is performed to identify suitable agents for treatment.
- Sensitivity testing is performed *in vitro* to assess the ability of an agent to inhibit the growth of an organism at concentrations that are likely to be found in vivo:
  - Disc diffusion testing and zone breakpoint diameters give some information about sensitivity to a particular antibiotic.
- More detailed testing involves assessing the minimum inhibitory concentration (MIC) or minimum bactericidal concentration (MBC) – the minimum concentration at which the inhibition of growth or death of the organism occurs respectively.

Antibiotic resistance

- Certain bacterial species are innately resistant to certain antibiotics.
- Other species have developed resistance under the selection pressure of antibiotic use:
  - Presence of an antibiotic that kills a large proportion of the bacterial population will lead to a proliferation of resistant mutant strains.

- Genetic resistance mechanisms are then passed on to subsequent genera-
  tions, and can be transferred between individuals and even between species.
- Several mechanisms may contribute to the development of resistance:
  - Inactivation by enzymes: Expression of enzymes that inactivate anti-
    biotics leads to resistance in many bacterial species (e.g. beta-lactamases).
  - Impaired access to target site: Structural change to pores in the bacte-
    rial cell outer membrane reduce the amount of antibiotic that enters
    the organism.
  - Change to target site: Alterations in the binding site of many antibiot-
    ics results in reduced effectiveness and resistance.

PHARMACOKINETIC CONSIDERATIONS

- Effective use of antibiotics relies on achieving concentrations that will kill
  or inhibit bacteria in infected tissues. This requires consideration of pharmacokinetic principles.

Absorption

- For antibiotics with high oral bioavailability (e.g. **amoxicillin, ciprofloxacin** and **clindamycin**), IV administration is only required if oral administration is not possible (for example, if patient is vomiting).
- Others (e.g. **cefepime**) require parenteral administration to achieve effective
  plasma levels, or are not absorbed orally (**gentamicin, piperacillin**).

MICRO-print
- **Vancomycin** has a poor oral bioavailability, but may be adminis-
  tered orally for a 'local' action within the gut in the treatment of
  Clostridium difficile infection.
- There are specific oral preparations, although commonly the IV
  preparation is administered orally or via NG tube (unlicensed).

Distribution

- Adequate penetration into the infected tissues is an important consideration
  in antibacterial selection:
  - Tissue penetration of many antibiotics improves when inflammation
    is present (for example, beta-lactams only achieve therapeutic levels
    within the CNS when meningeal inflammation is present).
- Organisms such as *Legionella pneumophilia* are intracellular and require
  agents that achieve high intracellular concentrations for treatment.

Metabolism

- Interactions with cytochrome P450 enzymes may lead to clinically
  significant drug interactions for some antibiotics (notably **ciprofloxacin,
  rifampicin** and the macrolides) (see Ch. 4, Section 4.2).

Drugs and practical prescribing

Elimination

- Most antibiotics are excreted in the urine, and renal impairment may require dose reduction or reduced dosing frequency.
- Agents that are eliminated unchanged in the urine are useful for urinary tract infections (e.g. nitrofurantoin).
- Excretion of active drug or metabolites into the bile occurs with many antibiotics and this is useful in biliary/enteric infections. Enterohepatic reabsorption may also increase useful half-life.
- Agents with a narrow therapeutic range (e.g. **gentamicin** and **vancomycin**) often require serum level monitoring (see Ch. 4, Section 4.2).

11.2 ANTIBIOTIC CLASSES

In the sections below, the following short-hand is used to describe the antibacterial spectrum of individual antibiotics:

- G+ve: Gram positive
- G−ve: Gram negative
- >: Excellent coverage
- <: Poor coverage

Bacteria may be classified as Gram positive or Gram negative. It is also useful to know which exist as intracellular organisms, as this factor effects their sensitivity to antibiotics. A list of commonly encountered bacteria can be found in Table 11.1.

MICRO-facts

Table 11.1 **Classification of bacteria**

GRAM POSITIVE	GRAM NEGATIVE	INTRACELLULAR ORGANISMS
Staphylococcus spp.	Coliforms	*Chlamydia* spp.
Streptococcus spp.	*Escherichia* spp.	*Mycoplasma* spp.
Enterococcus spp.	*Klebsiella* spp.	*Coxiella* spp.
Listeria spp.	*Salmonella* spp.	*Rickettsia* spp.
Bacillus spp.	*Shigella* spp.	*Treponema* spp.
Corynebacterium spp.	*Proteus* spp.	*Leptospira* spp.
Clostridium spp. (anaerobes)	*Haemophilus* spp.	
	Pseudomonas spp.	
	Neisseria spp.	
	Campylobacter spp.	
	Legionella spp.	
	Bacterioides spp. (anaerobes)	

BETA-LACTAMS

- Large group of antibacterial agents sharing a common beta-lactam ring in their molecular structure. Prototypical agent is **penicillin**.
- All beta-lactams exert their bacteriocidal effect by inhibiting a vital stage in bacterial cell wall synthesis, resulting in subsequent cell lysis.
- Main adverse effects are hypersensitivity reactions (see MICRO-facts below).

Penicillins
Examples
- **Benzylpenicillin (penicillin G)**
  - Spectrum:
    - G+ve (high *Streptococcus* spp. activity, but unstable to β-lactamase producers).
    - G−ve: >*Neisseria* spp., <*Haemophilus* spp; also active against spirochetes (treponema, leptospira).
  - Indications:
    - Endocarditis (plus gentamicin as empirical treatment).
    - Cellulitis (plus flucloxacillin 1 g IV 6 hourly).
    - Others: *Neisseria* spp. cover (meningitis, gonorrhoea).
  - Dosing: IV/IM 1.2–2.4 g 4–6 hourly depending on severity (high dose in endocarditis).
- **Phenoxymethylpenicillin (penicillin V)**
  - Spectrum: Mainly indicated in treatment of *Streptococcus* spp.
  - Indication: Tonsillitis.
    - Poor oral absorption limits use in other indications, must be taken on an empty stomach to optimize bioavailability.
  - Dosing: Oral 500 mg QDS (1 g if severe).

Beta-lactamase inhibitors and extended spectrum penicillins
These classes of antibacterial agents have increased the spectrum of activity of penicillins as a class by overcoming some of the bacterial defences.

Beta-lactamase inhibitors (and flucloxacillin)
- Numerous bacteria express beta-lactamase (penicillinase) enzymes which hydrolyze beta-lactam antibiotics, rendering them inactive.
- Addition of a beta-lactamase inhibitor increases the individual agents' spectrum of activity:
  - Beta-lactamase inhibitors: clavulanic acid, tazobactam and sulbactam.
  - They have no intrinsic antibacterial activity.
  - Inhibit bacterial beta-lactamases and prevent the breakdown of co-administered penicillins.
  - Examples include amoxicillin + clavulanic acid = co-amoxiclav.

- Flucloxacillin is chemically modified to infer resistance to breakdown by staphylococcal beta-lactamases.

Extended spectrum penicillins

- Modifications in chemical structure also increase the spectrum of antibacterial activity of agents:
  - Aminopenicillins such as **amoxicillin/ampicillin** have increased activity against G–ve bacteria due to better penetration of the outer membrane.
  - Anti-pseudomonal penicillins such as **ticaracillin** and **piperacillin** broad-spectrum penicillins, and are active against *Pseudomonas aeruginosa* (inherently resistant to multiple agents).
- These agents may also be used in combination with beta-lactamase inhibitors to increase the spectrum of activity (see examples below).

Examples

- **Flucloxacillin:**
  - Methicillin is the laboratory equivalent, methicillin-resistant *Staphylococcus aureus* (MRSA) implies resistance to flucloxacillin.
  - Spectrum: *Staphylococcus* spp. (penicillinase resistant)
  - Indications: Cellulitis/soft tissue infections (plus penicillin G 1.2 g 4 hourly); staphylococcal endocarditis (plus other agents in prosthetic valve); osteomyelitis (plus fusidic acid).
  - Dosing: Oral 250–500 mg 6 hourly; IM as oral, IV normally 500 mg–2 g 6 hourly
  - Poor oral absorption in the presence of food in the stomach, take on empty stomach.
- **Amoxicillin/ampicillin:**
  - Amoxicillin has better oral bioavailability.
  - Spectrum:
    - G+ve (β-lactamase sensitive).
    - >G–ve than benzylpenicillin; also *Listeria* spp.
  - Indications: Lower respiratory tract infection (LRTI)/community acquired pneumonia (CAP); urinary tract infection (UTI); otitis media; *Listeria* spp. infection (e.g. bacterial meningitis in >55 yrs/neonates).
  - Dosing: Oral: (amoxicillin) 250–500 mg 8 hourly; IM: 500 mg 8 hourly; IV: 500 mg 8 hourly–1 g 6 hourly.
- **Co-amoxiclav (amoxicillin + clavulanic acid, Augmentin®):**
  - Poor CSF penetration.
  - Spectrum: As amoxicillin, but β-lactamase resistance broadens spectrum; some anaerobe cover.
  - Indications: CAP (severe); hospital-acquired pneumonia (HAP), UTI (severe); animal bites; dental infection with spreading cellulitis
  - Dosing (mg as total drug combination): Oral: 375–625 mg 8 hourly; IV: 1.2 g 8 hourly

- **Piperacillin-tazobactam (Tazocin®):**
  - Piperacillin is unstable to extended spectrum beta lactamases and AmpC beta lactamases requiring co-administration with tazobactam.
  - Spectrum: G+ve (but β-lactamase sensitive) + *Haemophilus* spp. + *Neisseria* spp. Good *Pseudomonas* spp. cover.
  - Indications: Neutropenic sepsis (±gentamicin); HAP; *Pseudomonas* spp. infection, complicated intra-abdominal infections.
  - Dosing (grams as total drug combination): IV: 4.5 g 6–8 hourly.
- **Ticaracillin-clavulanic acid (Timentin®):**
  - Anti-pseudomonal, similar spectrum to piperacillin.

Cephalosporins

- Structurally related to penicillins with greater resistance to beta-lactamases (although many G–ve bacteria now produce beta-lactamases that degrade these agents).
- *Listeria* spp. are innately resistant and anaerobe cover is unreliable.
- Classified into generations, with more G–ve and less G+ve coverage in the higher generations.

First generation

- **Cefalexin:**
  - Oral agent with good concentrations in urine but less in other tissues.
  - Spectrum: G+ve (<*S. pneumoniae*) and <*E. coli*.
    - Not normally oral equivalent of IV cefuroxime when converting to oral preparations.
  - Indications: UTI (not first-line/severe); UTI prophylaxis.
  - Dosing: Oral, 250 mg 6 hourly or 500 mg 8–12 hourly.

Second generation

- **Cefuroxime:**
  - Parenteral agents with improved tissue concentrations and beta-lactamase resistance.
  - Spectrum: G+ve (good staphylococcal coverage); *H. influenza* + *E. coli*.
  - Indications: UTI (severe); biliary tract infection; abdominal infection/surgical prophylaxis (often with metronidazole); severe CAP in pen allergy (plus a macrolide).
  - Dosing: IV/(IM max 750 mg) 750 mg–1.5 g 8 hourly.

Third generation

- **Cefotaxime:**
  - Good tissue penetration including CNS, greater G–ve activity and less susceptibility to resistance mechanisms.

Drugs and practical prescribing

- Spectrum: G+ve and >G–ve than 1G agents (better *H. influenzae* + *S. pneumoniae* than ceftazidime).
- Indications: Bacterial meningitis; HAP.
- Dosing: IV/IM, 1 g 12 hourly increased to 8 g in four divided doses (severe, e.g. meningitis); max 12 g daily.
- **Ceftriaxone:**
  - Spectrum: Similar spectrum of activity and indications to cefotaxime; once daily dosing allows outpatient antibiotic treatment.
  - Dosing: IV/IM 1 g daily (max 4 g).
- **Ceftazidime**:
  - Good activity against *Pseudomonas* spp.
  - Spectrum: <G+ve and >G–ve than cefotaxime (including *P. aeruginosa*).
  - Indications: HAP; *Pseudomonas* spp. infections.
  - Dosing: IV/(IM max 1 g) 1 g 8 hourly; 2 g 8–12 hourly in severe.
- Some oral 3G agents are available (e.g. **cefixime**) with similar spectrum of activity to cefotaxime.

Advanced generations

- Fourth-generation (e.g. **cefipime**) and fifth-generation agents (**ceftaroline**) are now available with extended spectrum, including anti-pseudomonal and anti-MRSA activity.

Carbapenems

- Carbapenems (**meropenem, ertapenem, imipenem**) are beta-lactam agents with very broad spectrum of activity and stability to beta-lactamases (including extended-spectrum beta lactamases [ESBL] produced by some G–ve bacteria).
- Unfortunately several beta-lactamases are now prevalent that degrade carbapenems (e.g. carbapenemases).
- Carbapenems often represent the 'last line of defence' against resistant bacteria.

Examples

- **Meropenem (Meronem®):**
  - Spectrum: Almost all bacteria including ESBL producers (not MRSA).
  - Indications: Neutropenic sepsis (allografts); infections due to resistant organisms/clinical failure of empirical antibiotics.
  - Dosing: IV 500 mg–1 g 8 hourly.
- **Ertapenem (Invanz®):**
  - Spectrum: As meropenem (not *Pseudomonas* spp./*Acinetobacter* spp.)
  - Indications: CAP, abdominal/gynaecological infections due to resistant organisms.
  - Dosing: IV 1 g daily.

- **Imipenem/cilastatin (Primaxin®):**
  - Imipenem is enzymatically metabolized by the kidney. It is administered as a compound preparation with cilastatin to block renal metabolism.
  - Spectrum and indications: As meropenem.
  - Dosing: IV 500 mg–1 g 6 hourly.
- **Doripenem (Doribax®):**
  - Similar to meropenem.

Monobactams (mono-cyclic beta-lactam)

- **Aztreonam:**
  - Good activity against G−ve organisms (including *Pseudomonas* spp.) but no G+ve or anaerobe cover.
  - Dosing: IV 1–2 g 6–8 hourly; inhaled (in cystic fibrosis) 75 mg 8 hourly for 28 days.

MICRO-facts

Beta-lactam allergy and other adverse effects

- Hypersensitivity is the main adverse event associated with beta-lactams.
  - Up to 10% of individuals claim to have penicillin allergy but only 5–10% of these will have a reaction to an administered dose of penicillin.
  - The nature of claimed penicillin allergy should be carefully delineated and documented.
- Antibiotics often cause GI upset and patients may report this as 'allergy'.
- Anaphylaxis is extremely rare, occurring in around 0.05% of individuals.
  - The antigenic material is usually one or more metabolites, and cross-reactivity between individual agents and classes occurs:
  - All penicillins demonstrate cross-reactivity, so allergy to one agent will produce a reaction on exposure to another agent.
- There is some cross-reactivity with cephalosporins (around 8%) and carbapenems (around 10%) – these agents may be used if there is a history of minor penicillin allergy (rash), but avoided in cases of more severe allergy.
- Other adverse effects:
  - Interstitial nephritis: Penicillins/extended spectrum penicillins, cephalosprorins.
  - Seizures: Penicillins (at high doses).
  - Cholestasis/jaundice: Co-amoxiclav, flucloxacillin.

GLYCOPEPTIDES

- Intravenous agents only active against G+ve bacteria.
- Inhibit cell wall synthesis (earlier stage of synthesis than beta-lactams).
- Used in infections due to G+ve bacteria resistant to alternative agents (e.g. MRSA) and infections in patients with severe penicillin allergy (if other agents not suitable).
- Vancomycin requires therapeutic drug monitoring and many centres will produce their own guidelines.
- Monitoring is usually required after the third/fourth dose, or earlier in renal impairment (teicoplanin does not usually require monitoring unless toxicity or subtherapeutic levels are suspected).
- As time-dependent killing occurs peak concentrations are less of a concern and therefore avoidance of accumulation is main consideration (see MICRO-facts below).

Main adverse effects

- Ototoxicity: Dose dependent, occurs rarely with current preparations.
- Renal impairment: Especially if used with aminoglycosides (e.g. gentamicin).
- Red man syndrome: Rapid infusion of vancomycin (less than 1 hour) can cause severe flushing related to histamine release (less frequent with teicoplanin).

Examples

- **Vancomycin**
  - Spectrum: G+ve cocci (inc. MRSA), some vancomycin-resistant enterococci (VRE) are emerging.
  - Indications: Severe G+ve infection (endocarditis, MRSA infections); ORAL for *C. difficile* colitis.
  - Dosing: IV, 0.5–1 g 12 hourly.
    - Requires serum monitoring – pre-dose level 10–15 mg/L (15–20 mg/L in severe/less sensitive).
  - Not absorbed systemically following oral administration. May be used 'topically' for local actions via oral route (125 6 hourly for 10–14 days) for treatment of *C. difficile* colitis. The IV preparation will also not cross into the intestine from the plasma and is not suitable for treatment of this condition.
- **Teicoplanin**
  - Spectrum and indications: As for vancomycin.
  - Dosing: IV 400 mg 12 hourly for 3 doses then 200 mg daily (400 mg severe).

MICRO-facts

Vancomycin administration

- Due to time-dependant (not concentration dependant) killing, vancomycin may be administered as an infusion (e.g. in ITU settings).
- In renal failure, the appropriate dose for weight may be administered with levels checked subsequently.
- To avoid cumulative toxicity, then the next dose may be administered when the plasma concentration falls into pre-dose/trough range i.e. it is safe to give a first stat-dose irrespective of renal function provided levels will be subsequently checked.

MACROLIDES

- A group of agents that act by inhibiting bacterial protein synthesis.
- Binding to the 50S subunit of the bacterial ribosome prevents formation of initiation complexes and thus protein synthesis.
- Macrolides are initially bacteriostatic, becoming bacteriocidal at higher concentrations.
- They have intracellular antibacterial activity, making them useful against pathogens such as *Chlamydia* spp.

Adverse effects

- Gastrointestinal: Diarrhoea, colicky abdominal pain (prokinetic action on gut), nausea and vomiting are common with erythromycin and often lead to discontinuation – less common with newer agents.
- Acute cholestasis: Can occur with macrolides, likely a result of hypersensitivity.
- QT interval prolongation: Concurrent use with other agents that prolong the QT interval may result in arrhythmias (e.g. torsades de pointes or VF). Macrolides antibiotics inhibit cytochrome P450 enzymes resulting in multiple interactions and increased serum concentrations of numerous drugs (see Ch. 4, Section 4.2).

Examples

- **Erythromycin:**
    - Spectrum: Similar (not identical) to penicillin:
        - G+ve cocci (*Staphylococcus* spp. often resistant).
        - G−ve (not *Pseudomonas* spp./*Enterococcus* spp.).
        - Intracellular organisms.
    - Indications: CAP; skin/soft tissue infection; campylobacter enteritis.
    - Dosing: Oral/IV 250–500 mg 6 hourly; 500 mg–1 g 12 hourly.

- **Clarithromycin:**
  - Spectrum: Similar spectrum (plus *Haemophilus* spp.) and indications to erythromycin; better tolerated.
  - Dosing: Oral/IV 500 mg 12 hourly.
- **Azithromycin:**
  - Spectrum: As erythromycin (better *Chlamydia* spp. cover).
  - Indications: *Chlamydia* spp/genitourinary infections; CAP; otitis media; prophylactic treatment in COPD/bronchiectasis; typhoid; Lyme disease.
  - Dosing: Oral, 250–500 mg daily (250 mg 3× weekly in prophylaxis).
- **Telithromycin**
  - Spectrum: Similar to erythromycin.
  - Indications: Respiratory tract infections due to resistant organisms.
  - Dosing: Oral, 800 mg daily.

MICRO-print

- Macrolides are used in addition to broad spectrum penicillins in the treatment of severe community pneumonia.
- Their activity against intracellular organisms means that they broaden the spectrum of antibacterial cover to include atypical respiratory pathogens, including *Chlamydia* spp., *Legionella* spp. *Mycoplasma* spp. and *Coxiella* spp.
- Macrolides such as azithromycin and telithromycin also have some immunomodulatory activity, which is utilized in the management of chronic respiratory disorders such as cystic fibrosis.

TETRACYCLINES

- Bacteriostatic agents that inhibit bacterial protein synthesis by binding to 30S ribosomal subunit.
- Active against some G+ve bacteria (including some MRSA), some G–ve bacteria and intracellular organisms.
- Avoid in pregnancy and in children under 12 years of age as tetracyclines deposit in bones and teeth causing abnormal skeletal development and tooth discolouration.
- Excellent oral bioavailability.
- Milk- and calcium-containing preparations significantly reduce absorption.
- Demeclocycline used in treatment of SIADH as it inhibits action of ADH.
- Most common adverse effect is gastric irritation.

Examples

- **Doxycycline:**
  - Spectrum: G+ve (including most MRSA); <G–ve (*Neisseria* spp.); intracellular organisms.

- Indications: COPD; CAP/HAP; MRSA infection; UTI; malaria prophylaxis; infective endocarditis, *Chlamydia* spp./*rickettsia* spp. infection.
- Dosing: Oral, 100 mg daily (usually 200 mg loading dose).
- **Tetracycline/oxytetracycline:**
  - Spectrum: As doxycycline.
  - Indications: COPD exacerbations; acne (prolonged course); MRSA infection; *Chlamydia* spp. infection.
  - Dosing: Oral, 250–500 mg 8 hourly.
- **Lymecycline:**
  - Spectrum: As doxycycline.
  - Indications: Acne (prolonged course).
  - Dosing: Oral, 408 mg 12 hourly.

AMINOGLYCOSIDES

- Intravenous agents that are active mainly against G–ve bacteria (including *Pseudomonas* spp.), as well as being used synergistically with penicillins in G+ve infections.
- Act by binding to 30S subunit of bacterial ribosome, inhibiting protein synthesis.
- Exhibit concentration-dependant killing – increasing drug concentrations increase the proportion of bacteria killed.
- The significant toxicity of these agents means they have a narrow therapeutic range and require serum level monitoring.

MICRO-facts

Aminoglycoside dosing

- Traditionally administered in two or three daily doses, adjusted for weight and renal function (dosing intervals increased in renal impairment).
- Pre-dose (trough) and post-dose (peak) serum levels are measured around the third dose and determine the level and frequency of further dosing.
- **Once-daily dosing** is now used for most indications as it is more convenient and associated with a lower incidence of adverse effects, as it allows time for the drug to be washed out of the tissues.
- Most regimens are based upon the Hartford gentamicin regimen, with doses calculated using ideal body weight (IBW). It requires monitoring of serum levels 6–14 hours after the first dose, which predicts the trough levels. The subsequent dosing interval is adjusted according to a nomogram.
- Some situations are not suitable for once daily dosing, for example, endocarditis, burns, pregnancy, patients on dialysis or creatinine clearance (CrCl) <40mL/min, cystic fibrosis, CNS/ophthalmic infection.

Drugs and practical prescribing

Adverse effects

- Adverse effects are correlated to trough serum concentrations:
  - Nephrotoxicity: Commonly with gentamicin, especially if used concomitantly with other nephrotoxic agents. Usually reversible.
  - Ototoxicity: Usually irreversible damage to auditory vestibular apparatus, increased incidence with concomitant use of furosemide.

Examples

- **Gentamicin:**
  - Spectrum:
    - G−ve (inc. *Pseudomonas* spp.); synergism with penicillins against *Streptococcus* spp./*Staphylococcus* spp.
    - No G+ve cover when used alone.
  - Indications: Pyelonephritis; endocarditis (+benzylpenicillin); empirical therapy in severe infections (+ amoxicillin and metronidazole).
  - Dosing: IV multi dose: 1.5 mg/kg 8 hourly; once daily: 5–7 mg/kg; lower doses in synergy.
    - Multi dose serum levels: Pre/post dose around third dose – pre <2 mg/L, 1 h post 5–10 mg/L.
    - Once daily serum levels: 8 h post first dose 1.5–6 mg/L (further doses calculated using nomogram).
- **Tobramycin:**
  - Spectrum: Similar spectrum to gentamicin but better *Pseudomonas* spp. cover.
  - Indications: UTI; severe G−ve infections; nebulized in chronic *Pseudomonas* spp. infection in cystic fibrosis.
  - Dosing: IV multi dose: 1.5 mg/kg 8 hourly; once daily: 5–7 mg/kg.
    - Nebulized 300 mg 12 hourly for 28 days.
    - Serum levels monitoring as gentamicin.
- **Amikacin:**
  - Spectrum: As gentamicin.
  - Indications: Gentamicin-resistant G−ve infections.
  - Dosing: IV multi dose: 7.5 mg/kg 8–12 hourly; once daily: 15 mg/kg.
    - Serum levels: Multi dose: 1 h post <30 mg/L, pre <10 mg/L; OD: pre <5 mg/L.

QUINOLONES

- Broad spectrum agents that act by inhibition of bacterial DNA synthesis.
- Bind to DNA gyrase and topisomerase, preventing transcription of DNA.
- Excellent bioavailability means IV administration only required if impaired absorption/poor oral intake.

Adverse effects

- Tendon damage: Including rupture which may occur after cessation of treatment, discontinue if evidence of tendonitis.
- Prolonged QT interval:
  - Caution required in patients with risk factors for QT prolongation (moxifloxacin contraindicated).
  - Avoid concomitant use with other agents that may prolong QT interval (includes many drugs e.g. antidepressants, antipsychotics, macrolides).

Examples

- **Ciprofloxacin:**
  - Spectrum: G−ve (including *Pseudomonas* spp.); intracellular organisms.
  - Indications: UTI (resistant organisms); bacterial gastroenteritis; typhoid; genitourinary infection.
  - Dosing: Oral 250–750 mg 12 hourly; IV 400 mg q8–12h.
- **Levofloxacin:**
  - Spectrum: As ciprofloxacin; better G+ve cover (including *S. pneumoniae*).
  - Indications: COPD exacerbations; CAP; UTI.
  - Dosing: Oral/IV 250–500 mg daily.
- **Moxifloxacin**
  - Spectrum: As levofloxacin; useful antimycobacterial cover.
  - Indications: COPD exacerbations; CAP; skin/soft tissue infection; mycobacterial infection (second line).
  - Dosing: Oral/IV 400 mg daily.

MICRO-facts

Quinolone antibiotics should be avoided if possible in the hospital setting as they can predispose to nosocomial infection:
- Disruption of bowel flora can lead to *C. difficile* colitis.
- Excretion through skin kills normal skin commensals and leads to MRSA colonization.

OTHER ANTIBIOTICS

Metronidazole

- Nitroimidazole agent active against anaerobic bacteria. Also acts as a potent anti-protozoal agent (mainly active against gut protozoa).
- Disulfiram-like reaction may occur with alcohol causing severe vomiting.

Drugs and practical prescribing

- Indications: Abdominal infection/surgical prophylaxis; *C. difficile* infection; dental infection; giardiasis, amoebic infection.
- Dosing: Oral 400 mg 8 hourly; IV 500 mg 8 hourly; PR 1 g 12 hourly.

Clindamycin

- Inhibits bacterial protein synthesis. Active against G+ve (including some MRSA) and anaerobic organisms.
- Resistance to macrolides (e.g. erythromycin) usually infers resistance to clindamycin.
- Useful for skin/soft tissue infections in penicillin allergy as excellent bio-availability and skin/soft-tissue penetration.
- High risk of *C. difficile* colitis, especially if >60 yrs (discontinue if diarrhoea develops).
- Dosing: Oral 150–450 mg 6 hourly; IV/IM (deep) 0.6–2.7 g daily in 2–4 divided doses.

Chloramphenicol

- Bacteriostatic agent, inhibits bacterial protein synthesis. Broad spectrum, few innately resistant organisms.
- Commonly used for topical treatment of conjunctivitis.
- Rarely used systemically in developed countries due to high toxicity – occasionally used in meningitis, typhoid and neonatal sepsis.
- Adverse effects:
  - Myelosuppression: Occurs predictably after 1–2 weeks of treatment; usually reversible, may cause aplastic anaemia.
  - Grey baby syndrome: Accumulation may occur in neonates due to insufficient metabolic capacity with grey colouration, flaccidity and haemodynamic collapse. Serum level monitoring required.
- Dosing: Oral 12.5 mg/kg 6 hourly; IV/IM 500 mg 6 hourly.
  - Conjuctivitis (topical): Ointment QDS, eye drops 2 hourly initially and reduce according to symptoms, continue for 48 hours after symptoms stop.

Trimethoprim/co-trimoxazole

- Inhibits bacterial dihydrofolate reductase, preventing synthesis of folate (required for DNA synthesis).
- Active against some G–ve bacteria (not *Pseudomonas* spp.) including coliforms often implicated in UTI.
- Combined with sulfamethoxazole (**co-trimoxazole, Septrin®**) – broad spectrum antibacterial cover plus activity against *Pneumocystis jirovecii* and *Toxoplasma* spp.
- Greater toxicity than trimethoprim – risk of blood and skin disorders (including Stevens-Johnson syndrome).

- Adverse effects:
  - Mostly related to antifolate effect (anaemia/leucopenia/neutropenia) – can be reduced by co-administration of folic acid without affecting antimicrobial activity.
  - Small reduction in folate synthesis in human cells – avoid in pregnancy as may result in neural tube defects.
  - Hyperkalaemia also noted side effect.
- Dosing:
  - **Trimethoprim:** Oral 100 mg 12 hourly (usually three-day course for UTI).
  - **Co-trimoxazole:** Oral/IV 960 mg 12 hourly; *Pneumocystis jirovecii* pneumonia (PCP) treatment 120 mg/kg in 2–4 divided doses for 14–21 days; PCP prophylaxis 480–960 mg daily (or 960 mg alternate days)

Nitrofurantoin

- Rapidly absorbed and excreted into urine with almost no systemic effects.
- CrCl >60 mL/min required to achieve adequate urinary concentrations.
- G+/G−ve cover – may be used to treat UTI in pregnancy or severe penicillin allergy.
- Pulmonary fibrosis is important adverse effect – occurs after prolonged use.
- Dosing: Oral 50 mg 6 hourly.

Daptomycin (Cubicin®)

- Novel agent; binds to bacterial cell membranes and inhibits protein/RNA/DNA synthesis inducing cell death.
- Active against G+ve bacteria (including MRSA and some VRE) – indicated for treatment of resistant G+ve infections (for example, soft tissue infection, endocarditis).
- Main adverse effect: Muscle damage (including rhabdomyolysis) – requires monitoring of creatine kinase at least weekly.
- Dosing: IV 4–6 mg/kg daily.

Fusidic acid

- Narrow spectrum anti-staphylococcal agent that inhibits bacterial protein synthesis.
- Used in G+ve infections, especially penicillin-resistant staphylococci (e.g. staphylococcal osteomyelitis, endocarditis).
- Must be used in conjunction with a second anti-staphylococcal agent due to rapid development of resistance.
- Oral route only (tablets/suspension), IV form toxic.
- Dosing: Oral, 500 mg 8 hourly.

Linezolid (Zyvox®)

- First agent in a new antibiotic class (oxazolidinones).
- Acts by inhibiting bacterial protein synthesis (novel mechanism prevents cross resistance with other classes).
- Acts as an MAOI; therefore caution required with diet and other drug interactions (see Ch. 8, Section 8.2).
- Active against G+ve bacteria, including MRSA, usually reserved for severe infections resistant to alternative agents.
- Main adverse effects:
  - Haematological problems (anaemia/leucopenia/thrombocytopenia) – usually reversible.
  - Optic neuropathy after prolonged use (>28 days).
- Dosing: Oral/IV 600 mg 12 hourly.

ANTI-TUBERCULOUS AGENTS

- Active tuberculosis is initially treated with a combination of four agents – this ensures good anti-mycobacterial coverage against organisms of unknown sensitivity and prevents development of resistance.
- **Rifampicin (R):**
  - Inhibits bacterial/mycobacterial RNA synthesis
  - Also used for *Staphylococcal* spp./*Streptococcal* spp. infections (including endocarditis/MRSA infection, but not as monotherapy).
  - Powerful cytochrome P450 inducer – many drug interactions.
  - Adverse effects: Hepatotoxicity; red/orange discolouration of secretions; disseminated intravascular coagulation (DIC)/purpura.
  - Dosing: Oral/IV TB: <50 kg 450 mg daily; >50 kg 600 mg daily.
- **Isoniazid (H):**
  - Inhibits mycobacterial cell wall synthesis
  - Adverse effects: Hepatotoxicity; peripheral neuropathy (incidence reduced by administration of pyridoxine [vitamin B6]); blood disorders.
  - Dosing: Oral 300 mg daily.
- **Pyrazinamide (Z):**
  - Unknown mechanism of action; kills residual intracellular tubercule bacilli.
  - Adverse effects: Hepatotoxicity (including liver failure) and arthralgia.
  - Dosing: Oral <50 kg 1.5 g daily; >50 kg 2 g daily.
- **Ethambutol (E):**
  - Inhibits stage in mycobacterial cell wall synthesis.
  - Adverse effects: Optic neuropathy (requires pre-treatment testing of visual acuity).

- Dosing: Oral 15 mg/kg daily.
  - The first-line four-drug regimen (RHZE) may be reduced to isoniazid/rifampicin (RH) after two months in sensitive organisms, then continued for a further four months.
  - Fixed dose combination preparations are available:
    - **Rifinah®:** Isoniazid/rifampcin; also used in treatment of latent TB.
    - **Rifater®:** Isoniazid/rifampicin/pyrazinamide.
  - Supervised treatment may be required – three times weekly dosing.
  - Alternative second-line agents are used when resistance to first-line agents is present:
    - Injectable agents: streptomycin, capreomycin, amikacin.
    - Fluoroquinolones: moxifloxacin.
    - Oral agents: cycloserine, ethionamide, para-aminosalicylic acid (PAS).
    - New agents: bedaquiline, delamanid.

12 Antimicrobials II: Antivirals and antifungals

- In contrast to most antibacterial drugs, antiviral agents tend to be specific for the treatment of one family of virus.
- Doses are usually fixed and often used as fixed combinations with multiple anti-virals (for example, in HIV or hepatitis C).

12.1 ANTIRETROVIRALS

- Human immunodeficiency virus (HIV) infection is treated with a combination of antiretroviral agents known as highly active anti-retroviral therapy (HAART) (see Table 12.1).
- This is to ensure maximal suppression of viral replication and prevent the development of drug resistance.
- A first-line regimen in treatment-naïve patients usually consists of two NRTIs and an NNRTI.
- Other combinations and drug classes are used as second-line regimens and in treatment failures.

Table 12.1 **Antiretroviral drug combinations**

BRAND NAME	DRUG COMBINATION
Combivir®	Zidovudine (AZT) + Lamivudine (3TC)
Kivexa®	Abacavir (ABC) + Lamivudine (3TC)
Truvada®	Tenofovir (TDF) + Emtricatibine (FTC)
Trizivir®	Abacavir (ABC) + Zidovudine (AZT) + Lamivudine (3TC)
Atripla®	Tenofovir (TDF) + Emtricatibine (FTC) + Efavirenz (EFZ)
Eviplera®	Tenofovir (TDF) + Emtricatibine (FTC) + Rilpivirine
Keletra®	Lopinavir (LPV) + Ritonavir (RIT)
Triumeq®	Abacavir (ABC) + Lamivudine (3TC) + Dolutegravir

> ## MICRO-facts
>
> **Immune reconstitution inflammatory syndrome (IRIS)**
> - In advanced HIV infection, the immune system becomes weakened to the point where it cannot mount a response against invading pathogens.
> - After initiation of antiretroviral therapy, the improvement in immune system function may result in an overwhelming inflammatory reaction directed against opportunistic organisms.
>
> For this reason, initiation of antiretroviral treatment requires a careful assessment of the patient and liaison with specialists.

NUCLEOSIDE REVERSE TRANSCRIPTASE INHIBITORS (NRTIs)

Pharmacodynamics

- NRTIs act as nucleoside analogues to competitively inhibit HIV reverse transcriptase. This results in termination of DNA polymerization and prevents formation of HIV DNA from viral RNA.
- Two agents (a purine and a pyramidine analogue) form the 'backbone' of a HAART regimen. See MICRO-print below for fixed dose combinations.
- Lamivudine, emtricitabine and tenofovir are also effective in chronic hepatitis B virus (HBV) as well as in HIV infection.

Adverse effects

- Lipodystrophy (see MICRO-facts below)
- Lactic acidosis (due to inhibition of mitochondrial DNA polymerase)
- Hepatotoxicity
- Peripheral neuropathy
- Pancreatitis (ddI, d4T)
- Hypersensitivity (ABC – associated with HLA B57:01)
- Myelosuppression (AZT)

Examples

- **Zidovudine** (AZT)
- **Stavudine** (d4T)
- **Didanosine** (ddI)
- **Lamivudine** (3TC)
- **Abacavir** (ABC)
- **Emtricatibine** (FTC)
- **Tenofovir** (TDF)

MICRO-facts

Lipodystrophy

- The lipodystrophy syndrome is a collection of metabolic effects that are associated with many antiretroviral drugs, particularly nucleoside reverse transcriptase inhibitors and protease inhibitors.
- Features include insulin resistance, hyperlipidaemia and fat redistribution (especially with **zidovudine** and **stavudine**).
  - Stigma associated with fat redistribution may affect patient concordance with medication, and patients should be counselled.

NON-NUCLEOSIDE REVERSE TRANSCRIPTASE INHIBITORS (NNRTIs)

Pharmacodynamics

- NNRTIs non-competitively inhibit HIV reverse transcriptase by directly binding to the enzyme, preventing DNA polymerization. This prevents viral DNA formation and therefore further viral replication.
- Usually used with NRTIs in a first-line regimen
- Not effective against HIV-2

Adverse effects

- Hepatotoxicity (especially Nevirapine)
- Hypersensitivity

Examples

- **Efavirenz** (EFV)
- **Nevirapine** (NVP)
- **Etravarine** (ETR)
- **Rilpivirine**

PROTEASE INHIBITORS

Pharmacodynamics

- Protease inhibitors inhibit viral protease and prevent cleavage of viral proteins and virion assembly. This results in the production of non-infectious viral particles.
- Protease inhibitors often inhibit CYP3A4, with potential for significant drug interactions (increased serum levels of other drugs metabolized by this enzyme).

- **Ritonavir** acts as a particularly potent CYP inhibitor, and at low dose is used to boost the serum concentration of other protease inhibitors (available as fixed-dose combination with lopinavir).
- Used mainly in second-line regimens

Adverse effects

- Insulin resistance/diabetes (worsening control may be significant)
- Lipodystrophy (see MICRO-facts above)
- Lipid abnormalities

Examples

- **Saquinavir** (SAQ)
- **Lopinavir** (LPV)
- **Ritonavir** (RIT)
- **Atazanavir** (ATZ)
- **Darunavir** (DRV)
- **Fosamprenavir**
- **Indinavir**
- **Nelfinavir**
- **Tipranavir**

OTHER AGENTS

Integrase inhibitors

- HIV replicates by integrating its genetic material into the host DNA, using the host cellular apparatus to form new viral proteins.
- **Raltegravir** and **dolutegravir** inhibit HIV integrase activity, preventing insertion of viral genetic material into the host genome.
- Adverse effects:
  - Rash (may be severe, including SJS)
  - GI disturbance
  - Lipid abnormalities
- Lipodystrophy

Fusion inhibitors

- Entry of HIV into host cells requires fusion of viral and host cell membranes.
- **Enfurvitide** binds to the gp41 subunit of viral glycoprotein and prevents fusion of viral and host cell membranes.
- Adverse effects:
  - Hypersensitivity
  - Pancreatitis
  - Injection site reactions
- Only available as an injectable form

CCR5 receptor antagonists

- Entry of HIV into host cells requires interaction between host receptors and viral proteins.
- In CD4 receptor expressing cells, interactions with a co-receptor is required for viral entry, and tropism is the term used for the viral strain's ability to use these receptors.
- Two co-receptor subtypes exist:
  - CXCR4 tropism emerges in later disease.
  - CCR5 tropism is commonly expressed in early disease. It is this receptor on host immune cells that interacts with the viral gp120 protein and facilitates cell entry.
- **Maraviroc** binds to host cell CCR5 receptors, preventing viral cell entry.
- HIV may enter host cells via interaction with other receptors, in which case inhibition of host CCR5 will not prevent host cell infection.
- An HIV tropism assay is required to assess if Maraviroc will be effective.
- The main adverse effects are gastrointestinal disturbances.

Antiretroviral drug combinations

Many antiretroviral drugs that are commonly used together are available in fixed-dose combinations to reduce pill burden and improve compliance (Table 12.1).

- A common (and recommended in national guidelines) first-line regimen is TDF + FTC + EFZ.
- Other combinations such as ABC + 3TC + EFZ or TDF + FTC + ATZ/r are also widely used in certain circumstances.

12.2 OTHER ANTIVIRAL AGENTS

ACICLOVIR AND RELATED DRUGS

- **Aciclovir** is active against herpes simplex virus (HSV) and varicella zoster virus (VZV) with low toxicity due to preferential targeting of cells infected with the virus.
- It is selectively converted into an inactive nucleoside analogue by viral thymidine kinase.
- Subsequent incorporation into viral DNA complexes results in inhibition of viral DNA synthesis via premature chain termination.
- This prevents further viral replication, but does not eradicate viruses.
  - Treatment therefore should be started as early as possible and aims to reduce severity and duration of symptoms.
- Common uses include:
  - HSV:
    - Lips/eye: Topical therapy often appropriate (apply 5 times daily)

- Genital: Oral therapy normally sufficient
  ○ Typically 200 mg 5 times daily for 5 days
- Recurrence of infection or immunocompromised patients may require higher doses or longer duration of therapy.
- Severe infections (including encephalitis) require IV therapy.
- VZV:
  - Chickenpox: Neonates (IV), children (not normally required), adolescents and adults 40 mg/kg in four divided doses (normally 800 mg QDS)
  - Shingles: Dose as above
  - Neonates, nursing mothers, pregnant women and the immuno-compromised may require varicella-zoster immunoglobulin and specialist advice.
- Dose reduction is required in renal impairment, and the elderly are more susceptible to the neurological effects (see below).
- **Valaciclovir** is a prodrug of aciclovir that displays fewer adverse effects.
- **Famciclovir** is a prodrug of the topically applied aciclovir analogue, penciclovir.
- Adverse effects:
  - Acute kidney injury
  - Jaundice, hepatitis
  - Severe local inflammation on intravenous infusion
  - Photosensitivity, rash (including SJS with famciclovir)
  - Neurological effects: confusion, hallucinations, ataxia, convulsions

GANCICLOVIR AND DRUGS ACTIVE AGAINST CYTOMEGALOVIRUS (CMV)

- **Ganciclovir** and **valganciclovir**
  - Mechanism of action similar to aciclovir (active metabolite inhibits viral DNA polymerase), but much greater activity against CMV.
  - Valganciclovir is a prodrug of ganciclovir with reduced toxicity.
  - Adverse effects (significantly greater toxicity than aciclovir):
    - Myelosuppression (especially when used concurrently with zidovudine)
    - Rash
    - CNS toxicity
    - Retinal detachment (in CMV retinitis)
- **Cidofovir**
  - Acts as nucleotide analogue that is incorporated into viral DNA and prevents viral replication. Effective against most herpes viruses.
  - Adverse effects:
    - Nephrotoxicity
    - Eye disorders: iritis, uveitis

- **Foscarnet**
  - Inhibits viral DNA and RNA polymerase (also HIV reverse transcriptase). Active against most herpes viruses and some activity against HIV.
  - Highly toxic, adverse effects include:
    - Nephrotoxicity
    - Hypocalcaemia
    - Blood disorders (thrombocytopaenia, granulocytopaenia etc.)
    - Genital ulceration due to excretion in urine

OSELTAMIVIR AND ZANAMIVIR

- Active against influenza A and B viruses.
- They act via inhibition of viral neuraminidase, a glycoprotein required for viral replication.
- Zanamivir is only available as an inhaled preparation.
- Renally excreted, therefore may require dose adjustment
- Adverse effects:
  - **Oseltamivir:**
    - GI disturbance
    - Convulsions
    - Neuropsychiatric disorders
  - **Zanamivir:**
    - Rash
    - Bronchospasm

DRUGS USED IN VIRAL HEPATITIS

Hepatitis C

- **Interferon-alpha 2a/2b**
- Interferons are endogenous proteins that have immunomodulatory effects, particularly in the immune response to viral infection.
- They are used in the initial treatment of hepatitis C.
- Injectable only; used in combination with **ribavirin**.
- **Pegylated interferon-alpha:** Polyethylene glycol (PEG) is bound to interferon molecules to increase $T_{1/2}$ and serum concentrations. Improved efficacy.
  - Adverse effects:
    - Flu-like symptoms
    - Marrow suppression
    - Lipid abnormalities
    - May also cause depression
  - **Ribavirin**
    - Interferes with viral RNA synthesis by acting as a purine analogue. Also inhibits viral DNA production.

- Active against many viruses but licensed for use in HCV and respiratory syncytial virus (RSV)
- Inhaled and oral forms available
- Adverse effects:
  ○ Marked teratogenicity, and may remain in the body for up to 6 months. Must exclude pregnancy and both males and females should use contraception after administration.
  ○ Haemolytic anaemia
  ○ Rash (including SJS)
  ○ Pruritis
  ○ Depression
  ○ CNS toxicity

- **Telaprevir** and **Bocepravir**
  - Inhibit hepatitis C virus (HCV) protease and therefore prevent viral synthesis.
  - They are only effective in inhibition of hepatitis C virus genotype 1.
  - Used in combination with interferons and ribavirin, usually where first line treatment has failed.

Hepatitis B

- **Pegylated interferon-alpha** or **interferon-alpha** (see above) are indicated for initial treatment of chronic hepatitis B.
- Other initial options are **Entecavir** and **Telbivudine:** Nucleoside analogues that are incorporated into viral DNA and inhibit viral enzymes.
- Subsequent options include **Adefovir** (nucleotide analogue).

12.3 ANTIFUNGAL DRUGS

TRIAZOLES

- Selectively inhibit fungal cell CYP450 enzymes, reducing ergosterol production (required for cell wall synthesis) and leading to cell death.
- Indications:
  - Candidiasis, aspergillosis, cryptococcosis, histoplasmosis, dermatophytoses, pityriasis versicolor
- Adverse effects:
  - GI upset
  - Hepatotoxicity, including hepatitis
- Interactions: Enzyme inhibition leads to increased levels of many drugs (including warfarin).
- Examples:
  - **Fluconazole (Diflucan®)** (good oral bioavailability and CNS penetration)

- **Itraconazole**
- **Posaconazole**
- **Voriconazole**

IMIDAZOLES

- Mechanism of action similar to triazoles, but non-selectively inhibit CYP450 enzymes, leading to drug interactions.
- The oral license for ketoconazole was recently withdrawn due to hepatotoxicity so they are now only available in topical preparations.
- Indicated in dermatophytoses and candidiasis
  - Examples:
    - **Clotrimazole**
      - Multiple preparations including 1% (common skin infections, including tinea pedis etc.) and 2% creams (vaginal candidiasis), pessaries (vaginal candidiasis).
    - **Miconazole:** Oral gel available for oral candidiasis
    - Others: **Ketoconazole, econazole, tioconazole**
- Adverse effects as triazoles

POLYENES

- **Amphotericin** binds to ergosterol in fungal cell membranes, forming pores that allow movement of intracellular contents, resulting in cell death.
  - Some binding to cholesterol in human cell walls occurs, resulting in toxicity.
    - Available as IV preparations.
    - Lipid formulations also available. **Liposomal amphotericin (Abelcet® and AmBisome®)** have significantly lower toxicity compared to non-lipid preparations, but a higher cost.
  - Indications:
    - Invasive candidiasis, aspergillosis, cryptococcosis, histoplasmosis, blastomycosis
  - Adverse effects:
    - Infusion reactions: fever, vomiting, spasms, hypotension
    - Administered as slow infusion to reduce initial toxicity
      - Nephrotoxicity
      - Hepatotoxicity
      - Anaemia
      - Hypersensitivity
    - Anaphylaxis may occur: test dose required (1 mg over 20–30 min then normal dosing)

Drugs and practical prescribing

OTHER AGENTS

- **Caspofungin**
  - Fungicidal activity through inhibition of fungal cell wall protein synthesis
  - Indications: Invasive candidasis and aspergillosis; empirial antifungal therapy in neutropenia
  - IV form only
- **Griseofulvin**
  - Is incorporated into keratin and prevents fungal growth affecting skin and hair.
  - Main adverse effects are hypersensitivity reactions.
- **Flucytosine**
  - Is effective in the treatment of cryptococcosis, metabolites inhibit fungal cell RNA and DNA synthesis. Synergism with amphotericin occurs.
  - Bone marrow suppression and colitis are important adverse effects.
  - Monitoring required: LFTs, U+E and FBC weekly (blood dyscrasias, hepatotoxicity)
  - Dose according to plasma flucytosine concentration in renal impairment
- **Terbinafine**
  - Is incorporated into keratin and impairs fungal metabolism, active against dermatophytoses.
  - Used where topical therapy failed – drug of choice in fungal nail infections.

13 Musculoskeletal and metabolic drugs

13.1 CALCIUM AND BONE METABOLISM

GENERAL PRINCIPLES

- Bone pathologies are intrinsically related to bone metabolism and calcium homeostasis.
- Accordingly, the therapeutics of these diseases predominantly affect these two physiological pathways.
- Bone metabolism (or remodelling) is a dynamic process which at a cellular level is regulated by two classes of cells:
  - Osteoblasts: Secrete osteoid (type I collagen) to form a matrix, and regulate its calcium and phosphate based mineralization.
  - Osteoclasts: Mediate bone resorption, mobilizing these minerals from bone tissue into the extracellular fluids, ultimately affecting their serum levels.
- Calcium metabolism is regulated by three major factors:
  - PTH (parathyroid hormone):
  - Release stimulated by low calcium levels.
  - Increases serum calcium concentrations by:
    - Increasing bone resorption through indirect osteoclast stimulation.
    - Increasing renal tubular reabsorption of calcium and reducing reabsorption of phosphate.
    - Enhancing renal activation of vitamin D.
  - Vitamin D:
    - Inactive cholecalciferol undergoes two stage activation.
    - It is first metabolized in the liver to 25-hydroxycholecalciferol (calcidiol) and subsequently activated by the kidney into the active form, 1,25-dihydroxycholecalciferol (calcitriol).
  - Increases serum calcium levels through stimulation of intestinal absorption and bone resorption.
  - Calcitonin: Effects are the opposite of PTH.

MICRO-facts

Hypercalcaemia

- Hypercalcaemia may require urgent medical attention. Corrected Ca^{2+} levels >3.5 mmol/L are associated with QT shortening and arrhythmias.
- Rehydration with normal saline is first line therapy.
- Subsequently bisphosphonates such as pamidronate or zolendronate may be used.
- Clinical effects not seen for around 24 hours and maximally at around 5 days.
- **Calcitonin** and loop diuretics (e.g. **furosemide**) may also be considered. **Cinacalcet** is used in renal disease.

BISPHOSPHONATES

- Bisphosphonates decrease osteoclastic bone resorption and associated loss of bone mass.
- Used in pathologies associated with bone fragility and hypercalcaemia.
- Licensing and indications vary with individual drugs due to differing evidence bases.

Pharmacodynamics

- Bisphosphonates adsorb onto hydroxyapatite crystals of the bone preventing osteoclast mediated resorption with no direct effect on bone formation.

Pharmacokinetics

- Absorption:
- Bisphosphonates have very low bioavailability when given orally (often <1%).

MICRO-print

Bisphosphonates and food

- Bioavailability is further and significantly decreased in the presence of stomach contents.
- Adherence to consumption before food (particularly chelating agents such as milk [calcium] and iron preparations) is essential to ensure adequate absorption for clinical effect.

Indications

- Product dependant (see individual drug profiles)
- Generally as a class, bisphosphonates are used in osteoporosis, Paget's disease, hypercalcaemia of malignancy, bone pain and other complications of skeletal metastases.

Cautions and contraindications

- Gastric and oesophageal disease (risk of oesophageal ulceration with oral preparations – see below)
- Hypocalcaemia, vitamin D deficiency and osteomalacia
- Renal impairment (may require dose adjustment)
- Dental care and hygiene (risk of osteonecrosis of jaw)

Adverse effects

- GI: Gastritis/PUD, oesophageal reactions (oral preparations), other GI disturbance
- Metabolic: Hypocalcaemia, hypophosphataemia
- Musculoskeletal: Atypical femoral fractures
- Others: Flu-like symptoms, rarely osteonecrosis of the jaw (see above), blood dyscrasias

Important interactions

- Chelating agents (Ca^{2+}, iron, antacids): significantly reduce oral bioavailability

Examples

- **Alendronic acid (Fosamax®)**/once weekly
  - Osteoporosis: 10 mg OD or 70 mg weekly, PO
  - With **colecalciferol (Fosavance®)**
- **Risedronate sodium (Actonel®)**/once a week
  - Osteoporosis: 5 mg OD, or 35 mg weekly, PO
  - Paget's disease: 30 mg, OD, PO
  - With **calcium carbonate and colecalciferol (Actonel® Combi)**
- **Zolendronic acid**
  - **Zometa®:** Hypercalcaemia of malignancy, IV
  - **Aclasta®:** Paget's disease of bone, IV
- **Ibandronic acid**
  - **Bonviva®:** Osteoporosis, oral (monthly), IV (3 monthly)
  - **Bondronat®:** Hypercalcaemia, bony metastasis
- Others: **disodium pamidronate (Aredia Dry Powder®)** (IV – used in acute hypercalcaemia), **disodium etidronate (Didronel®)**/PMO (cyclically administered with calcium supplements – reduces concordance), **sodium clodronate (Bonefos®, Clasteon®, Loron 520)**

Special requirements

- Patients must be counselled on the following when prescribed oral preparations:
  - Take more than 30 minutes before food (see pharmacokinetics).
  - Take with a glass of water and sit/stand for 30 minutes after (reduces risk of oesophageal ulceration).

> **MICRO-print**
> **Monitoring with bisphosphonates**
> - Electrolytes including calcium and phosphate should be monitored initially, around a month after starting and at routine follow up.
> - Renal function should be monitored due to potential toxicity.
> - Serum alkaline phosphatase is measured in Paget's disease of bone as a marker of osteoclastic activity.

CALCITONIN AND PARATHYROID HORMONES

Calcitonin

- Calcitonin has effects which are opposite to that of parathyroid hormone.
- Synthetic/recombinant salmon calcitonin (**salcatonin [Miacalcic®]**) is available as injection or nasal spray, and is used in hypercalcaemia of malignancy, Paget's disease of bone, osteoporosis and immobility induced bone loss.

Parathyroid hormone and related drugs

- Human recombinant parathyroid hormone **Preotact®** is available for osteoporosis.
- **Teriparatide (Forsteo®)** is a recombinant fragment of PTH licensed for osteoporosis, but is also indicated for men at risk of fractures.
- **Cinacalcet (Mimpara®)** is a calcimimetic, which acts on the parathyroid gland reducing PTH output by 'mimicking' the negative feedback mechanism. It is used in hypercalcaemia and secondary hyperparathyroidism associated with end stage renal disease.

STRONTIUM RANELATE

- **Strontium ranelate (Protelos®)** is used in osteoporosis to rebalance bone turnover in favour of bone formation.
- Increases osteoblast precursor formation and reduces osteoclastic bone resorption.

13.2 NEUROMUSCULAR DRUGS

SKELETAL MUSCLE RELAXANTS

- These drugs are used primarily to treat chronic spasticity associated with neurological conditions including multiple sclerosis and spinal cord lesions.
- Benzodiazapines such as **diazepam** are also occasionally used in the chronic setting. This class of drugs is also sometimes used in acute muscle spasms, such as those associated with minor injuries (see Ch. 8, Section 8.5).

Baclofen

- Baclofen is a GABA derivative that binds to and activates $GABA_B$ receptors which results in inhibition of neurotransmission both centrally and at spinal level.
- This results in a reduction in muscle tone and hypotonia. Sedation is also common.
- Other less common neurological effects include psychiatric disturbances and seizures.
- Caution in many neurological conditions:
  - Epilepsy (possible decrease seizure threshold)
  - Parkinson's disease (increased risk psychiatric disturbances)
  - Stroke (low efficacy, possibly reduced seizure threshold)
- Indications: Chronic severe spasticity (usually in multiple sclerosis or spinal cord damage).
  - May be used via intrathecal pump to increase CNS delivery.
- Dosing: Start low (5 mg TDS, Orally) and increase slowly to avoid adverse effects.
- Warn patients about sedation and driving.
- Enhances hypotensive and sedative effects of other medications.
- Abrupt cessation may precipitate side effects. Ensure therapy is continued as prescribed.

Dantrolene

- Peripheral action on skeletal muscle through reduction in excitation-contraction coupling.
- Fewer central effects compared to baclofen, benzodiazepines and tizanidine.
- Decreases intracellular Ca^{2+} available for muscle contraction, mechanism not fully elucidated.
- Potentially hepatotoxic therefore contraindicated in hepatic disease, warn patients of symptoms and check liver function at follow ups.
- Indications: Chronic severe spasticity, malignant hyperpyrexia (further information in MOTM anaesthesia).
- Dosing: Start low (25 mg OD) and increase slowly to avoid adverse effects.
  - IV preparation used in malignant hyperpyrexia.
- Warn patients about sedation and driving.

Tizanidine

- Centrally acting muscle relaxant. Agonism of pre-synaptic α_2 receptors ultimately reducing NMDA mediated neurotransmission at spinal interneurons.
- This results in reduced muscle tone with reduction in spasm and clonus.
- Indications: Chronic severe spasticity.

- Potentially hepatotoxic, take caution in hepatic disease. Monitor liver function for 4–6 months following initiation of treatment.
- Warn patients about sedation and driving.
- Enhances hypotensive effects of other medications.
- Abrupt cessation may precipitate rebound tachycardia and hypertension. Withdraw slowly.

ANTICHOLINESTERASES (ACETYL CHOLINESTERASE INHIBITORS)

- These agents act to enhance the effects of acetylcholine (ACh) at nicotinic receptors at the neuromuscular junction (NMJ).
- They are used in the treatment of myasthenia gravis and to reverse the effects of non-depolarizing muscle relaxants (atracurium, vercuronium – further information in MOTM Anaesthesia).

Pharmacodynamics

- Competitively inhibit the action of the enzyme acetylcholinesterase (AChE) leading to increased ACh concentrations at the synaptic cleft.
- This prolongs and intensifies ACh effect at the neuromuscular junction (nicotinic receptors).
- They also, however, act at both subclasses of acetylcholine receptor (nicotinic and muscarinic) in the autonomic nervous system which results in the 'cholinergic adverse effects' (see below).
- In myasthenia gravis, antibodies to ACh receptors impair action potential transmission across the NMJ. This is partially overcome by increasing the amount of available ACh.
- Non-depolarizing muscle relaxants competitively inhibit ACh receptors (selective nicotinic action). Increasing the concentration of ACh in the NMJ displaces the muscle relaxant reversing its effects.
- Myaesthenia gravis.
- **Edrophonium** used for diagnosis (**Tensilon®** test).
- Reversal of non-depolarizing muscle relaxant (edrophonium/neostigmine) – see below.

Contraindications

- Urinary retention
- Intestinal obstruction

Cautions

- Related to parasympathetic receptor activation
- Asthma (bronchoconstriction)
- Bradycardia/arrhythmias/recent MI
- Parkinsonism

Adverse effects

- Cholinergic crisis:
    - AChE overdose may result in complete inhibition of ACh breakdown, resulting in an excessive neuromuscular block.
    - Muscle paralysis and respiratory failure result.
    - Treatment is with anticholinergic drugs (for example, atropine).
- Muscarinic effects: Hypersalivation, lacrimation, diarrhoea/incontinence, urination, meiosis, bradycardia, bronchoconstriction/bronchial secretions, hypotension, muscle weakness.

Important interactions

- Aminoglycosides and polymixin antibiotics (occasionally used in cystic fibrosis) antagonize the effects of anticholinesterases (may result in neuromuscular blockade even in normal NMJ).

Examples

- **Edrophonium:** Must be administered where resuscitation facilities are available due to risk of severe cholinergic reactions.
- **Neostigmine:**
    - Oral for myasthenia gravis treatment, short duration of action.
    - IV for reversal of muscle relaxation in combination with anticholinergic (e.g. glycopyrronium) to counter autonomic cholinergic effects.
- **Pyridostigmine:** Orally for myasthenia gravis, less effective than neostigmine, but lower muscarinic effects and longer duration of action.

QUININE

- Mainly used for its antimalarial activity, quinine sulphate is also used off-license for the treatment of nocturnal cramps.
- It prolongs the refractory period of the motor end plate, reducing muscle cramps in around 25% of ambulatory patients.
- Its use, however, is limited by its toxicity and it is not recommended first line.

Adverse effects

- Cinchonism: Flushing, tinnitus, blurred vision, hearing impairment, nausea/vomiting. Rare with oral treatment.
- Toxicity: May cause cardiac arrhythmias (long QTc, ventricular arrhythmias), seizures, acute renal failure, blindness, electrolyte and glycaemic derangement. Death is not uncommon.

Dosing

- **Quinine sulphate:** Normally 300 mg at night

Drugs and practical prescribing

13.3 GOUT

TREATMENT OF ACUTE GOUT

General principles

- Acute attacks of gout are treated with anti-inflammatory agents, typically NSAIDs (see Ch. 10, Section 10.3).
- Colchicine is used in situations where NSAIDs are contra-indicated or there is a high-risk of adverse effects.
- These agents do not alter uric acid metabolism.
- Corticosteroids (oral or intra-articular) and **Canakinumab** (recombinant monoclonal antibody) may be considered if the above are contraindicated or have failed to treat symptoms.

Colchicine

Pharmacodynamics

- Prevents microtubule assembly by binding to tubulin. This inhibits mitosis and neutrophil activity, producing an anti-inflammatory effect but no other analgesic effects.

Indications

- Acute gout
- Prophylaxis of gout
- Familial Mediterranean fever

Cautions

- Gastrointestinal disease

Contraindications

- Blood disorders
- Pregnancy

Adverse effects

- Gastrointestinal disturbance: Especially diarrhoea at high doses, may limit use.
- Others (high dose): Renal and hepatic impairment, rash, GI haemorrhage

Important interactions

- Drugs that inhibit hepatic CYP450 enzymes may increase risk of adverse effects.

> ## MICRO-facts
>
> ### Colchicine dosing, adverse effects and interactions
>
> - Diarrhoea limits dose. Maximum course is 6 mg prescribed as 500 micrograms 2–4 times daily.
> - Long-term treatment is associated with bone marrow suppression. Patients should be warned of signs of neutropenia and thrombocytopenia.
> - Colchicine is subject to a multitude of bi-directional CYP450 enzyme interactions. These should be considered prior to prescribing.

CONTROL OF CHRONIC GOUT

General principles

- These agents have effects on uric acid metabolism and are used in the prophylaxis of gout and the treatment of hyperuricaemia.
- Drugs used for the long-term prophylaxis of gout should not be started during an acute attack, as they may exacerbate and prolong the acute phase.

Allopurinol

Pharmacodynamics

- Allopurinol acts as a purine analogue and competitively inhibits the action of xanthine oxidase, reducing the synthesis of uric acid and lowering serum uric acid concentrations.
- Xanthine oxidase is the final enzyme in the metabolic pathway of purine metabolism that converts multiple metabolites to uric acid, which can be excreted.

Pharmacokinetics

- Allopurinol itself is metabolized by xanthine oxidase, and the product of this metabolism also inhibits the enzyme.

Indications

- Prophylaxis of gout
- Prophylaxis/treatment of uric acid renal stones
- Prophylaxis of chemotherapy-induced hyperuricaemia
- Treatment of hyperuricaemia in tumour lysis syndrome (now rarely used)

Cautions

- NSAID (or colchicine) therapy should be administered for a month following initiation of allopurinol to prevent the precipitation of an acute attack.

- Due to the side effect profile, start at low dose and titrate according to uric acid levels.
- Renal impairment: Maximum dose 100 mg OD. In severe impairment monitor plasma-oxipurinol concentration.

Contraindications

- Treatment of acute gout.
- Allopurinol initiation during an acute attack of gout can exacerbate symptoms, and initial therapy should be delayed for weeks after acute attack.

Adverse effects

- Rash/hypersensitivity reactions: Including severe skin reactions resembling TEN/SJS (relatively high incidence), vasculitis, hepatitis, seizures.
- Bone marrow suppression: Including aplastic anaemia.

Important interactions

- Allopurinol inhibits metabolism of purine analogues including 6-mercaptapurine and azathioprine – dose reduction required to prevent toxicity.

MICRO-print

Several other agents alter uric acid metabolism.

Probenicid

- Acts as a uricosuric agent, reducing the reabsorption of uric acid in the proximal tubule of the kidney and increasing excretion.
- High urinary concentrations of uric acid increase risk of stone formation.
- Probenicid also reduces the renal elimination of penicillin increasing serum penicillin levels. It is occasionally used as such in treatment of syphilis and actinomycosis.

Febuxostat

- New agent that non-competitively inhibits xanthine oxidase, reducing synthesis of uric acid. Limited to use in patients who cannot tolerate allopurinol therapy.
- NSAIDs should be administered for six months following initiation of treatment to avoid precipitating an attack of acute gout.

Sulphinpyrazone

- A uricosuric agent that is rarely used for prophylaxis of gout.

---

14 Prescribing anticoagulants

14.1 ANTICOAGULATION

BLOOD COAGULATION CASCADE

See Fig. 14.1.

WARFARIN

Pharmacodynamics

- Warfarin (and other coumarin anticoagulants) act by inhibiting the production of activated vitamin K-dependent clotting factors (factors II, VII, IX, X; Fig. 14.1).
- These clotting factors are activated by carboxylation by gamma-glutamate carboxylase (GGC), which in turn requires cyclical vitamin K metabolite production for activation.
- This cyclical reaction requires the enzyme vitamin K epoxide reductase (VKER) for continuation of the activation loop.
- VKER is inhibited by warfarin (see Fig. 14.2).
- Following warfarin administration there is consequently a net reduction in activation of the vitamin K dependent clotting factors.
- The anticoagulant effect of warfarin is due to the replacement of active clotting factors with their inactive counterparts, and the rate at which this occurs is dependent on the half-life of these active clotting factors in the circulation:
  - Factor VII: 6 h, factor IX: 24 h, factor X: 40 h, factor II: 60 h
  - Thus an initial anticoagulant effect (and increase in the INR) occurs after 6–8 h as active factor VII is replaced by the inactive form.
  - Full anticoagulation does not occur until factor II levels have dropped significantly (after 3–4 days).
- The effects of warfarin may be reversed by administering vitamin K (phytomenadione).

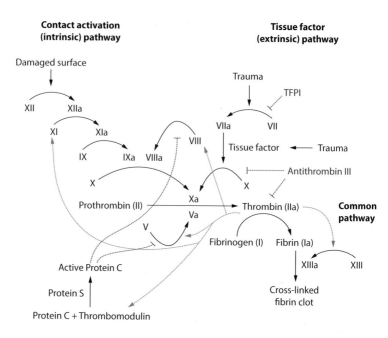

Fig. 14.1 The coagulation cascade showing actions of anticoagulant agents. (Reproduced with kind permission from the author Joe Dunckley, *More in-depth version of the coagulation cascade*, 2007: Creative Commons BY-SA 3.0.)

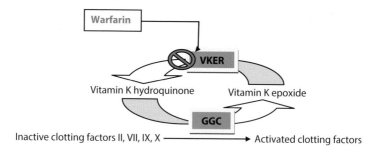

Fig. 14.2 Warfarin and vitamin K dependent clotting factor activation.

MICRO-print

International Normalised Ratio (INR)

- Warfarin anticoagulant properties are measured using the INR.
- The INR is a standardization of the ratio of the patient's prothrombin time to that of a normal control sample.

continued...

continued...

- Due to the differences between analytical reagents used in different labs, manufacturers assign a number (ISI value) to each batch of reagent that denotes how the reagent compares to an international standard.
- The prothrombin ratio is then raised to the power of the reagents ISI value to give a standardized measure of anticoagulation:

$$INR = \{PT_{patient}/PT_{control}\}^{ISI}$$

MICRO-facts

- By the same mechanism as outlined above, warfarin also reduces the production of active forms of protein C and protein S, which usually act to inhibit coagulation.
- This leads to an initially prothrombotic state when warfarin therapy is started. Accordingly, alternative anticoagulation (e.g. heparin) is also required during this period.

Pharmacokinetics

- Absorption: 100% oral bioavailability.
- Metabolism: Mainly hepatic to inactive metabolites.
- Distribution/elimination:
  - Small volume of distribution as highly bound to albumin.
  - Half-life of 40 h, renal excretion of metabolites.

Indications

- Venous thromboembolism (VTE): Target INR 2.5.
  - DVT: Normally 3 months if precipitated by reversible cause.
  - PE: Normally 6 months if precipitated by reversible cause.
  - Also indicated in venous sinus thrombosis.
  - Recurrent VTE in the absence of reversible causes often requires life-long therapy. Recurrence on warfarin mandates INR target 3.5.
- Other indications: Target INT 2.5.
  - AF, inherited thrombophilia, cardioversion or pulmonary hypertension.
- Replacement cardiac valves:
  - Tissue prosthetic valve (target INR 2.5 – usually short term).
  - Mechanical (target INR 3–3.5 dependent on type).

Adverse effects

- Bleeding: Spontaneous or due to minimal trauma. This may be massive and life threatening.

Drugs and practical prescribing

- Teratogenicity:
  - Warfarin crosses the placenta freely and may cause haemorrhage in the foetus.
  - It may also cause abnormal bone formation resulting in birth defects.
  - Greatest risk in first and third trimesters, although it should be avoided throughout pregnancy.
- Skin necrosis:
  - Rare but severe complication with necrosis of cutaneous tissue that may occur within the first few weeks of warfarin therapy.
  - The risk is greatest in those with protein C deficiency.

Important interactions

Warfarin has many clinically important drug interactions, resulting in either increased or reduced anticoagulant effect.

- Increased effect:
  - Displacement of warfarin from albumin binding sites: NSAIDs, hypoglycaemics, metronidazole, co-trimoxazole, macrolides, ampicillin, cephalosporins.
  - Inhibition of hepatic enzymes which metabolize warfarin: Acute alcohol excess, amiodarone, chloramphenicol, cimetidine, statins (not pravastatin), ketoconazole.
  - Reduced clotting factor production: Aspirin (high dose).
  - Reduced vitamin K synthesis: third generation cephalosporins.
- Reduced effect:
  - Induction of hepatic enzymes: Barbiturates, phenytoin, carbamazepine, rifampicin, OCP.
  - Reduced intestinal absorption: cholestyramine.
- Increased clotting factor activation: vitamin K (including dietary).

MICRO-facts

Managing interactions with warfarin
- If an interacting drug will be used for less than 5 days, often no dosage change is necessary. Omission of one day of warfarin dosage may be prudent with known potentiating drugs.
- Where interacting drugs are used, or if they are stopped it is recommended that the INR is checked after 3–5 days.

MICRO-reference
National Institute for Health and Clinical Excellence. *Anticoagulation-oral, Scenario: warfarin.* Clinical Knowledge Summaries. London, UK: NICE CKS, 2013. Available from: http://cks.nice.org.uk/anticoagulation-oral#!scenario:3 (accessed March 21, 2014).

Monitoring

- Anticoagulation with warfarin is monitored using the INR.
- Once stable, the INR may be measured monthly, and dosing requirements for the following weeks can be calculated.

Initiation of treatment

- As discussed above, a dose of warfarin will not begin to exert an anticoagulant effect until 6–8 hours post-administration, and the full effect will not be evident for 3–4 days.
- Thus, dose changes will not be reflected by changes in the INR for several days.
- Due to the long half-life of warfarin, it may take several weeks for plasma levels to reach steady state after initiation of treatment. For this reason, loading doses are usually given (especially in cases of acute thrombosis).
- The INR should be checked on day 1 (before initiation of treatment) and daily until stable (usually 4–5 days).

Rapid anticoagulation

See Fig. 14.3.

- Loading doses used where there is need to rapidly increase INR (e.g. treatment of VTE).
- Local protocols apply and are usually based upon modifications of the Fennerty regimen. For example:
  - Day 1: If INR <1.4 prescribe 10 mg (unless higher risk of overcoagulation)
    - Smaller loading doses (normally 5 mg) required in:
      - ○ Elderly patients.
      - ○ Liver/heart failure.
      - ○ Concomitant use of drugs that enhance anticoagulant effect of warfarin (see above).
  - Day 2 onwards: Doses based upon INR results as per local policy.
- Warfarin initially has a prothrombotic effect (see above). Alternative anticoagulation (usually with heparin) should be continued during the initiation of treatment until the INR is above 2.0 for two consecutive days.

Drugs and practical prescribing

STHFT Warfarin Treatment Management Guidelines

A. General Guidance on Initiating Warfarin (cross through dosing table below if using slow start regimen).

- Ensure baseline bloods (full blood count, liver function tests, urea and electrolytes, coagulation screen and baseline INR) are satisfactory before commencing warfarin.
- Explain to the patient the indication for warfarin treatment, risks and benefits.
- **Continue dalteparin for minimum of 5 days and until INR is greater than 2 for 2 consecutive days.**
- **Measure INR daily when <u>initiating</u> warfarin treatment.**
- NB The INR is not accurate if the APTT ratio is greater than 4.0 whilst on unfractionated heparin.

Day	*Patients aged under 65		**Patients aged 65 or over	
	INR (In Morning)	Warfarin Dose (mg) (In Evening)	INR (In Morning)	Warfarin Dose (mg) (In Evening)
1(Pre-treatment baseline)	Less than 1.4	10	Less than 1.4	10
2 If INR greater then 1.8, patient may be warfarin sensitive. Monitor frequently.	Less than 1.8	10	Less than 1.8	5
	1.8 – 2.0	1	1.8 – 2.0	1
	Greater than 2.0	0	Greater than 2.0	0
3	Less than 2.0	10	Less than 2.0	5
	2.0 – 2.2	5	2.0 – 2.2	4
	2.3 – 2.5	4	2.3 – 2.5	4
	2.6 – 2.9	3	2.6 – 2.9	3
	3.0 – 3.2	2	3.0 – 3.2	2
	3.3 – 3.5	1	3.3 – 3.5	1
	Greater than 3.5	0	Greater than 3.5	0
4	Less than 1.4	Greater than 8	Less than 1.4	Greater than 7
	1.4 – 1.5		1.4 – 1.5	7
	1.6 – 1.7	8	1.6 – 1.7	6
	1.8 – 1.9	7	1.8 – 1.9	5
	2.0 – 2.3	6	2.0 – 2.3	4
	2.4 – 3.0	5	2.4 – 3.0	3
	3.1 – 4.0	4	3.1 – 4.0	2
	Greater than 4.0	3	Greater than 4.0	1
		Omit dose until INR is 3.0 or under		0
				0
After day 4	Use clinical judgement		Use clinical judgement	

*Modified from British Society for Haematology Guidelines on Oral Anticoagulation: Third Edition. *Br J Haematology* 1998; **101**: 374–87 and Fennerty et al. *British Medical Journal* 1988; **297**: 1285–8.
Modified from Gedge et al., *Age and Ageing* 2000; **29: 31–34.

Fig. 14.3 General guidance for initiating warfarin therapy. (Permissions granted by Sheffield Teaching Hospitals Foundation Trust.)

Slow anticoagulation

- For some indications (such as AF) warfarin therapy may be initiated more slowly, possibly in an outpatient setting.
- In these situations, smaller loading doses (2–5 mg) are used to achieve the target INR over 1–2 weeks.
- This usually avoids overshooting the target INR.

Bridging protocols

- These protocols are typically used when warfarin must be stopped prior to elective surgery.
- Local protocols are commonly available and are based upon British Committee for Standards in Haematology guidance.
- Typically patients are classified into three to four levels of risk; for example:
  - Low risk: Non-valvular AF with no previous history of stroke, VTE over three months previously.
  - Intermediate risk: Valvular AF or recent VTE (less than three months).
  - High risk: Very recent VTE (less than six weeks), mechanical valve replacement.
- Pre-op: Stop warfarin five days before an operation and cover with low molecular weight heparin (LMWH).
  - Low/intermediate risk: prophylactic dose.
  - Intermediate/high risk: treatment dose.
- Day of surgery: Take INR pre-operatively, if greater than 1.5 give 1 mg IV vitamin K.
- Post-op: If no contraindication/bleeding risk start:
  - LMWH 6–8 h post op (prophylactic dose).
  - Restart warfarin at normal maintenance dose day 1 post-op, with risk determined LMWH cover until INR greater than 2 for two consecutive occasions.
- Note: For insertion or removal of epidurals there is increased risk associated with anticoagulation. Seek expert advice.

Overdose/overtreatment

- Over-anticoagulation (INR above target range) may result in bleeding, which may be severe and life-threatening.
- Management depends on the INR and the presence and severity of bleeding (Fig. 14.4):
  - Vitamin K_1 is also known as phytomenadione.
- High dose vitamin K_1 (e.g. 10 mg) should be avoided as the very long half-life may make re-anticoagulation difficult. This dose is normally used in pathological coagulopathy (e.g. secondary to hepatic disease).

Avoiding prescribing errors

- Errors in warfarin prescribing commonly result in harm to patients, and great care must be taken to avoid over- or under-anticoagulation.
- The INR must always be known before initiation of warfarin therapy.
- In cases where a patient on long-term warfarin is acutely admitted, the INR should be checked prior to prescribing further warfarin doses as intercurrent illness, other drugs and patient factors (i.e. unintentional overdose) can affect the level of anticoagulation.

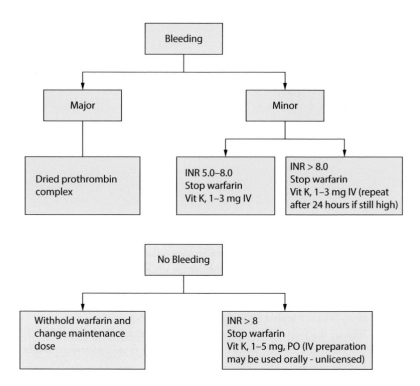

Fig. 14.4 Management of over-anticoagulation and reversal indications for warfarin. Local protocols may apply. (British Journal of Haematology Guidance and Joint Formulary Committee, *British National Formulary* (online), London: BMJ Group and Pharmaceutical Press, http://www.medicinescomplete.com, Oral anticoagulants, accessed on December 20, 2013.)

- Sudden large dose changes should be avoided, as this can result in unpredictable changes in the INR.
- When making dose adjustments it is always helpful to review the INR trend and recent dose changes, whilst remembering the time lag for warfarin's effect.

> **MICRO-reference**
> Keeling D, Baglin T, Tait C, et al. British Committee for Standards in Haematology. Guidelines on oral anticoagulation with warfarin, 4th edition. *British Journal of Haematology* 2011 Aug; 154(3): 311–324.

THE HEPARINS

General principles and pharmacodynamics

- Heparin acts by potentiating the effects of antithrombin III, an endogenous protein with anticoagulant properties:
  - Antithrombin III usually acts by binding to factors IIa, IXa and Xa, rendering them inactive. This process is usually very slow.
  - Heparin binds to antithrombin III and induces a confirmational change that increases the rate at which it interacts with these factors.
  - Once antithrombin III has bound to the relevant factor, heparin is released to bind another antithrombin III molecule.
  - The rate of deactivation of these important clotting factors is thus hugely increased, preventing progression to the common coagulation pathway and clot formation, and so producing an anticoagulant effect.
- Heparin is available as either unfractionated heparin (UFH) or low molecular weight heparin (LMWH):
  - Unfractionated heparin produces a marked decrease in the concentrations of thrombin (factor IIa) and factor Xa.
  - LMWH is produced from short chain fragments of heparin and has mainly anti-Xa activity.

Low molecular weight heparins

- LMWH is usually chosen in preference to UFH for prophylaxis of VTE due to ease of administration, prolonged duration of action, and lower risk of heparin-induced thrombocytopaenia (HIT).
- No monitoring is required allowing for greater ease of administration over unfractionated heparin (see below).
- Due to accumulation in renal impairment, a reduction in dose or avoidance of use is required with significant renal impairment. UFH may be a better alternative in these patients.

Pharmacokinetics

- Distribution/elimination:
  - Small Vd, renal elimination of metabolites.
  - Plasma $t_{1/2}$ 4–6 h, peak anti-Xa activity after 4–6 h, anti-Xa activity detectable for ~24 h .

Indications

- Prophylaxis of VTE
- Treatment of VTE and acute coronary syndromes

Drugs and practical prescribing

Examples

- **Enoxaparin.**
  - Prophylactic: 40 mg OD (20 mg OD if CrCl <30 mL/min).
  - Therapeutic: 1 mg/kg BD (ACS) or 1.5 mg/kg OD (VTE).
- **Dalteparin:** Prophylaxis usually 5000 units OD, treatment dose is weight based.
- **Tinzaparin:** Prophylactic and therapeutic doses weight based – see BNF.

Unfractionated heparin (UFH)

- Unfractionated heparin allows rapid anticoagulation and rapid reversal (either by stopping the infusion or by administering protamine).
- This is useful in situations where anticoagulation requirements may change rapidly (for example, peri-operatively, in cardiopulmonary bypass/haemodialysis circuits).
- It is also used in renal impairment where use of LMWH is contraindicated.

MICRO-print

Protamine

- In certain cases (for example, acute haemorrhage or cardiopulmonary bypass), rapid reversal of anticoagulation with heparin is required.
- Protamine is used to bind heparin forming an inactive complex.
- 100 units of heparin are bound by 1 mg of protamine, so to reverse a 5000 unit bolus of heparin would require 50 mg protamine.
- Protamine is less effective at reversing the effects of LMWH.

Pharmacokinetics

- Absorption: Usually administered intravenously; bioavailability after subcutaneous administration is dose dependant (usually less than LMWH)
- Metabolism: Hepatic
- Elimination:
  - Biphasic elimination – rapid initial clearance by saturable binding to reticuloendothelial cells and macrophages (zero order kinetics), followed by slower renal elimination of hepatic metabolites
  - Half-life is thus dose dependent, around 30 min at therapeutic doses

Indications

- Prophylaxis and treatment of VTE.
- Treatment of arterial thrombosis.
- Anticoagulation of extracorporeal circuits (cardiopulmonary bypass, haemodialysis etc.).

Initiation of treatment and dosing
- Initial bolus of 5000 units (or 75 units/kg) as loading dose.
- Omit if already on alternative anticoagulation or high risk of bleeding (e.g. significant post-surgical risk).
- Dosing is weight based – usually 15–25 units/kg/h initially, approximately 1500 units/h (may be administered as 50000 units made up to 50 mL with 0.9% NaCl infused at 1.5 mL/h via infusion pump).

Monitoring
- UFH is monitored using the activated partial thromboplastin time (APTT) ratio (the ratio of the test APTT to that of a control – there is no standardization protocol as with INR).
- The target APTT ratio is usually around 1.5–2.5 but varies between labs.
- After initiation of heparin therapy, the APTT ratio should be checked after 6 h, then 6 h after dose changes (sooner if a significantly out of range and a large dose change made or later if APTT ratio is stable and no dose change made).

Adverse effects (both UFH and LMWH)
- Bleeding: Can largely be avoided by careful administration and monitoring.
- Heparin induced thrombocytopaenia (HIT):
  - Severe thrombocytopaenia occurs in up to 5% of patients on heparin (less often with LMWH) due to an antibody-mediated response.
  - HIT should be suspected in any patient on heparin with a greater than 50% fall in platelet count or new thrombosis.
  - Most commonly develops after 5–10 days. Discuss with a haemotologist and switch to alternative anticoagulation with a thrombin or factor Xa inhibitor.
  - FBC should be monitored for those on LMWH for greater than 4 days.
- Hyperkalaemia: Due to inhibition of aldosterone secretion. Check U+E's before prescribing and at 7 days. Will need repeating if prolonged therapy.

MICRO-print

Heparin induced thrombocytopaenia
- Heparin forms complexes with a protein on the surface of platelets called platelet factor 4 (PF4).
- IgG antibodies are directed against this complex, which then forms cross links with antibody receptors on adjacent platelets.
- This causes activation and aggregation of platelets and clot formation.
- Increased generation of thrombin also contributes to the hyper-coaguable state which leads to venous and arterial thrombosis despite of the thrombocytopenia.

- Osteoporosis:
  - Long-term treatment may cause a decrease in bone mineral density (BMD) resulting in pathological fractures.
  - The risk is lower with LMWH, but may be significant when used throughout pregnancy.

Fondaparinux

- Synthetic pentasaccharide sequence (similar to sequence within heparin) that inhibits factor Xa via its interaction with antithrombin III
- Fondaparinux has no effect on thrombin, unlike unfractionated heparin.
- Essentially a very low molecular weight heparin that may avoid being targeted by anti-PF4-complex IgG and has therefore been proposed as a treatment for HIT.
- Administered subcutaneously with a half-life of ~20 hours that allows once-daily dosing.
- Renal elimination.
- Licensed for prophylaxis and treatment of VTE and in ACS.
- Main adverse effect is bleeding, low risk of HIT, does not usually require monitoring.
- Dosing:
  - VTE prophylaxis: 2.5 mg SC OD.
  - Treatment of VTE: 2.5 mg OD for >30 days (superficial vein thrombosis); 7.5 mg OD (adjusted according to weight) until oral anticoagulation adequate (DVT/PE)
  - UA/NSTEMI: 2.5 mg OD for 8 days (or until hospital discharge if sooner)
  - STEMI: 2.5 mg IV on first day, then 2.5 mg SC OD for 8 days

DIRECT FACTOR Xa INHIBITORS

- These drugs directly inhibit factor Xa, preventing progression to the common coagulation pathway and generation of thrombin (no direct effect on thrombin).
- They are orally active, and unlike the vitamin K-antagonists do not require any monitoring.
- Bleeding, either due to overtreatment, overdose or concomitant use of medications that increase the effect of the drug is the main adverse effect.
  - There are no available antidotes at present.
- Important interactions: Not affected to same extent as warfarin by hepatic enzyme induction and inhibition, although azole antifungals (for example, ketoconazole, itraconazole) and protease inhibitors increase anticoagulant effect.
- **Rivaroxaban:** Currently licensed in the UK for stroke prevention in non-valvular atrial fibrillation (20 mg OD), treatment of VTE (15 mg OD) and

prevention of VTE in patients undergoing major hip or knee surgery (10 mg OD – starting 6–10 hours post-surgery for 2/52 knee, 5/52 hip).

- **Apixiban:** Currently licensed in stroke prevention in non-valvular atrial fibrillation (5 mg BD, 2.5 mg BD <60 kg or elderly) and prophylaxis in orthopaedic surgery (2.5 mg BD, starting 12–24 h post-surgery).

OTHER ANTICOAGULANTS

Direct thrombin inhibitors

- **Lepirudin:** Derived from hirudin, an anticoagulant protein produced by leeches. Directly inhibits action of thrombin (independent from antithrombin). Used for anticoagulation in patients with HIT. Monitored using the APTT.
- **Bivalirudin:** Short-acting agent licensed for use in percutaneous coronary intervention and ACS.
- **Dabigatran:** Oral once daily thrombin inhibitor licensed for prevention of VTE after major hip and knee surgery. Does not require monitoring, main side effect is haemorrhage.

Heparinoids

- **Danaparoid:** Contains various glycosaminoglycans derived from heparin, and is administered subcutaneously or intravenously. Used as prophylaxis for VTE in orthopaedic surgery and also treatment of VTE in patients with HIT (provided no cross reactivity).

Prescribing of fluids

15.1 INTRAVENOUS FLUIDS, INFUSIONS AND ELECTROLYTES

FLUID COMPARTMENTS AND DAILY REQUIREMENTS

Fluid compartments

- The body is roughly 60% water by mass, which equates to around 42 litres in a 70-kg man.
- Fluid in the body is separated into several compartments, which have differing compositions:
    - Intracellular compartment (around 28 L): Main cation is potassium (150 mmol/L).
    - Extracellular compartment (around 14 L): Main cation is sodium (140 mmol/L), main anion is chloride (110 mmol/L). Further divided into:
        - Interstital compartment (around 11 L): Accumulation of fluid in interstitum produces oedema.
        - Intravascular compartment (around 3 L): With cellular components form/s the total circulating volume of around 5 L.
- A 'third space' is often mentioned – this describes any space (or potential space) in which fluid may be sequestered (e.g. pleura, peritoneum or retroperitoneum).
- Water can move freely between the compartments according to osmotic and oncotic gradients.
- If water is administered into the intravascular compartment, it will rapidly equilibrate throughout the total body fluid compartments, leaving only a small fraction in the intravascular compartment.
- Replacement fluids are formulated with additives to target replacement fluid volume in the desired compartment (see Fig. 15.1 and individual intravenous fluids below).

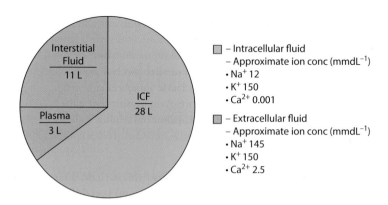

Fig. 15.1 Approximate fluid content per compartment as proportion of total body fluid in 70 kg man.

Daily fluid and electrolyte requirements

- In health, fluid balance is maintained by the body's response to sodium concentration:
    - Elevated sodium concentration leads to increased release of antidiuretic hormone (ADH) that reduces water excretion (resulting in dilution of body fluid).
    - Reduced sodium concentration suppresses ADH release and so water excretion is relatively increased.
- Daily fluid requirements (in health) reflect the balance between input and output:
    - Input: ~2500 mL (oral fluid intake: 1500 mL; food: ~1000 mL).
    - Output:
        - Urine 1500 mL.
        - GI tract 200 mL (fluid secretion by the gut totals up to 6 L daily but almost all is reabsorbed in health. Ion constituent broadly similar to that of ECF – Fig. 15.1).
        - Insensible losses (skin, respiratory tract) 800 mL.
- Daily electrolyte requirements are as follows (main source is food):
    - Sodium: 130–150 mmol (approximately 2 mmol/kg).
    - Chloride: 130–150 mmol.
    - Potassium: 60–70 mmol (approximately 1 mmol/kg).
- Any disease process that alters input or output may result in fluid and electrolyte imbalance:
    - Decreased input: Nausea/vomiting, inadequate fluids/iatrogenic fluid restriction; reduced patient drive to drink; upper GI obstruction.
    - Increased input: Psychogenic polydipsia; iatrogenic (over administration of IV fluids – commonly seen in hospital practice).

- Decreased output: Renal failure.
- Increased output:
  - Losses through normal mechanisms: Vomiting, diarrhoea, increased insensible losses (e.g. fever), diabetes insipidus, iatrogenic (e.g. excess diuretic).
  - Losses through other mechanisms: Haemorrhage, burns, surgical drains, third space losses.

FORMULATED INTRAVENOUS FLUIDS

- Fluids formulated for intravenous infusion are divided into crystalloid and colloid groups based on their composition.
- There has been much debate over the relative benefits of colloids and crystalloids, but current opinion is that with regard to fluid resuscitation:
  - Colloids confer no therapeutic benefit over crystalloids.
  - Are generally more expensive.
  - Carry a greater risk of hypersensitivity reactions compared to crystalloids.

Crystalloids

- Contain water and electrolytes or glucose (small particles).
- Tonicity relative to plasma varies between formulations.

Hypotonic (and relatively hypotonic)

- Water and glucose (dextrose): The glucose is rapidly metabolized and the water quickly equilibrates between all compartments therefore not suitable for resuscitation:
  - 5% glucose (dextrose):
    - Used for maintenance fluid, excess can produce hyponatraemia.
    - Slightly hypotonic, used to replace total body water in dehydration. Also used in sliding scale in diabetes.
    - Potassium may be added (see MICRO-facts box below).
    - Constituent: 50 g dextrose/L; osmolarity 271 mOsm/L.
  - 0.18% NaCl + 4% dextrose (commonly referred to as 'dextrose saline').
    - Slightly hypotonic. Suitable to replace intracellular fluid loss in dehydration. May be used as part of daily maintenance therapy provided sodium is provided elsewhere.
    - Constituents: sodium 31 mmol/L, dextrose 40 g/L; osmolarity 271 mOsm/L.
  - Others:
    - 0.18% and 0.45% NaCl (fifth and half-saline): These hypotonic solutions contain lower concentrations of sodium than 0.9% saline. Occasionally used in hypernatraemia (under senior advice only), not for maintenance therapy.

Isotonic

- Isotonic: Contain electrolytes in similar concentration to plasma; said to be 'physiological' and used for maintenance fluids as well as replacement and resuscitation.
    - **0.9% NaCl** (also known as '0.9% saline'):
        - May be used for fluid resuscitation where blood not required and maintenance therapy to provide appropriate daily sodium requirements (see below).
        - Excess use may produce hyperchloraemic acidosis and may lead to hypokalaemia (as below).
- Constituents: Na^+ 154 mmol/L and Cl^- 154 mmol/L (one litre provides daily adult requirements of Na^+ and Cl^-); osmolality 308 mOsm/L.

MICRO-facts

Addition of potassium to fluids

- Addition of potassium chloride to fluids is often appropriate in order to ensure adequate daily requirements are met (approx. 1 mmol/kg).
- It is commonly added to both NaCl 0.9%, dextrose 5% and 0.18% NaCl + dextrose 4% (dextrose saline). It may also be seen added to dextrose 10% in sliding scale regimens.
- Pre-made bags with potassium 20 and 40 mmol/L are commonly available, more concentrated solutions may be found but are not recommended in routine practice due to risk of rapid administration of potassium, and caustic nature causing thrombophlebitis.
- In critical care/anaesthesia concentrated potassium may be used through central lines with careful cardiac monitoring.

- **Hartmann's solution:**
    - Most closely resembles plasma composition.
    - Appropriate for replacement of plasma volume.
    - Lower chloride concentration may reduce likelihood of hyperchloraemic acidosis in comparison to 0.9% saline.
    - Composition: Na^+ 131 mmol/L, Cl^- 111 mmol/L, lactate 29 mmol/L, K^+ 5 mmol/L, Ca^{2+} 2 mmol/L, 279 mOsm/L.
- **Lactated Ringer's solution** and **Plasma-lyte** are similar to Hartmann's (electrolyte composition differs slightly).

Hypertonic

Should not be administered rapidly into small veins as hypertonicity may damage red blood cells.

- **Dextrose:**
  - 10%, 20% and 50% solutions are available.
  - May be used for treatment of hypoglycaemia or as part of sliding scale regimens.
- **NaCl:**
  - Hypertonic electrolyte concentrations (1.8%, 3% saline), occasionally used with senior input in the treatment of hyponatraemia.
  - Used occasionally as volume expanders as administration of hypertonic fluid will draw water into extracellular space from the intracellular space along the osmotic gradient (1 L of 3% saline expands volume by ~2.5 L).
  - However, likely to cause depletion of cellular water if insufficient isotonic fluids used (only use under specialist supervision).

MICRO-facts

Crystalloids in common use
- Dextrose
  - 5% (50 g/L).
    - Osmolarity 271 mOsm/L.
    - Used in maintenance therapy and rehydration.
  - 10%, 20% and 50%.
    - Osmolarities relatively increased from 5%.
    - Used in hypoglycaemia and sliding scale regimens.
- Dextrose 4%/sodium chloride 0.18%
  - Sodium 31 mmol/L, dextrose 40 g/L; osmolarity 271 mOsm/L.
  - Used in maintenance therapy and rehydration.
- Sodium chloride 0.9%.
  - Na^+ 154 mmol/L and Cl^- 154 mmol/L; osmolality 308 mOsm/L; used in maintenance therapy and fluid resuscitation.
- Hartmann's solutions (or similar)
  - Composition: Na^+ 131 mmol/L, Cl^- 111 mmol/L, lactate 29 mmol/L, K^+ 5 mmol/L, Ca^{2+} 2 mmol/L; 279 mOsm/L.
  - Most appropriate for replacement of plasma volume

Colloids

- Solutions containing large molecules (usually synthetic) such as starch or gelatin.
- These large molecules do not leave the intravascular space as readily as electrolytes and so water is held intravascularly by osmotic forces.
- Often used for fluid resuscitation as produce rapid volume expansion, although there is no evidence to suggest they are any better than crystalloids such as Hartmann's or NaCl 0.9%.

Drugs and practical prescribing

- Often expensive and the synthetic components can induce hypersensitivity reactions (including anaphylaxis).
- Usually contain similar concentrations of sodium to 0.9% saline.
- Examples: **Pentastarch, Volulyte®, Gelofusine®, Volplex®.**

FLUID PRESCRIBING

- When prescribing intravenous fluids there are several important considerations:
  - Is intravenous fluid really required? If the patient can eat and drink adequately and no additional fluid losses are ongoing, maintenance fluids may not be needed.
  - What is the patient's current fluid status?
    - Euvolaemic, hypervolaemic or hypovolaemic. A thorough assessment of the patient's volume status should be performed prior to prescribing any fluid.
    - Examination includes skin turgor, mucus membranes, jugular venous pressure (JVP), peripheral oedema, pulmonary oedema and heart sounds (third i.e. gallop rhythm).
    - Measured variables include heart rate, blood pressure, urine output (normal 0.5–1 mL/kg/h), urea and creatinine concentration.
  - Are there any ongoing losses that will affect fluid balance? See above.
  - Are there any electrolyte abnormalities that need correction?
    - Recent U+Es should be checked to guide any electrolyte administration (e.g. potassium) and to ensure that any abnormalities will not be exacerbated by administration of a particular fluid.
    - Consider body fluid losses, for example, small bowel secretions contain ion content similar to ECF (see Fig. 15.1), and gastric secretions contain varying but significant amount of sodium, 10–20 mmol/L of potassium and high concentrations of H^+ ions.
  - Are there any factors that may make the patient prone to rapid fluid overload?
    - Heart failure
    - Renal failure
    - Hypoalbuminaemia

Maintenance fluids

- Describes maintenance of normal daily fluid input when oral intake is not possible/desirable (e.g. peri-operatively, aspiration risk, fasting/nil by mouth).
- Normal daily fluid and electrolyte requirements are detailed above.
- Attention must be paid to fluid status and the rate of fluid administration adjusted accordingly.

Drugs and practical prescribing

MICRO-facts

Innumerate maintenance regimens may be appropriate, and the following example regimen meets the requirements of maintenance therapy for a standard adult (70 kg), taking into account daily sodium and potassium requirements. However, prescribing fluids must be individualized and based upon a thorough assessment of the patient.

- 1L *5% glucose* + KCl 20 mmol over 10 h
- 1L *0.9% NaCl* + KCl 20 mmol over 10 h
- 1L *5% glucose* + KCl 20 mmol over 10 h

Fluid replacement

- If there have been fluid losses additional to physiological output, there will be a total body water deficit.
- Where there have been excess losses (or fluid loss is ongoing), replacement fluid must be administered in addition to maintenance requirements.
- It may be possible to make up for additional fluid losses by increasing oral intake, but often intravenous replacement is required (especially if fluid losses are significant).

MICRO-facts

Fluid status assessment (tennis score system)
- This system is applicable in blood loss (trauma) and hypovolaemia from fluid loss.
- It serves only to guide initial therapy by emphasizing pathophysiological responses to shock.
- It is also known as the 'tennis' system as the percentage loss parameters are similar to tennis scores.
- The volumes are for a 70-kg adult patient.
- *Class 1:* 10–15% blood volume loss: (750 mL)
  - Physiological compensation and no clinical changes appear.
- *Class 2:* 15–30% blood volume loss: (750–1500 mL)
  - Postural hypotension, generalized vasoconstriction, oliguria 20–30 mL/h.
- *Class 3:* 30–40% blood volume loss: (1500–2000 mL)
  - Hypotension, tachycardia >120, tachypnoea, oliguria <20 mL/h, confusion.
- *Class 4:* 40% blood volume loss: (>2000 mL)
  - Marked hypotension, tachycardia and tachypnoea. Anuria, patient is comatose.

> **MICRO-reference**
>
> ACS Committee on trauma. *Advanced Trauma Life Support, Student Course Manual,* 9th edition. Chicago: American College of Surgeons; 2012.

- Fluid replacement to correct the fluid deficit should be administered in addition to maintenance requirements over 12–24 h.
- The rate of fluid administration depends on the degree of volume depletion and the clinical state of the patient. If the patient is haemodynamically compromised (class 3 to 4 shock) then immediate resuscitation is appropriate (as below).

Resuscitation

- Where fluid depletion is severe enough to produce a clinical state of shock, urgent fluid resuscitation is required.
  - The exception to this rule is in cardiogenic shock, where additional fluid is likely to be harmful as the hypotension is not due to hypovolaemia but secondary to insufficient cardiac output.
  - Caution should also be applied in neurogenic shock, where reduced vascular tone leads to vasodilation below the site of injury and a relative hypovolaemia. Fluids play some role in resuscitation, but inotropic support may be required.
- Rapid infusion of a suitable fluid is required to restore an adequate circulating volume:
  - Crystalloid or colloid may be administered as a 'fluid challenge':
    - 250-mL boluses of fluid given using three-way tap or pressure bag.
    - Gauge response to fluid resuscitation (i.e. reduction in tachycardia and normalization of blood pressure).
- If the cause of shock is blood loss then transfusion and/or surgical intervention should be considered.
- If a fluid challenge is effective, further fluid should be given to replace the volume deficit and return haemodynamic parameters towards normal.
- If it is not effective, repeat boluses may be used up to 2 L provided the patient will tolerate this volume (i.e. heart failure). During this time the differential diagnosis should also be considered and senior assistance requested.

MICRO-facts

In a fluid resuscitation situation crystalloids (usually 0.9% saline or Hartmann's solution) are preferred for fluid replacement of intravascular volume. Dextrose solutions would be distributed between all compartments of total body water, leaving only a small percentage in the intravascular space (see Fig. 15.1).

ELECTROLYTE DISTURBANCES

- The list below gives a brief outline of clinical features, causes and management of the common electrolyte disturbances, with prescribing advice where appropriate. Use local policies where they apply.
- The management of all electrolyte disturbances must include treatment of the underlying cause.

Potassium

Hyperkalaemia

Causes

- Renal impairment; potassium-sparing diuretics; ACE inhibitors, Addison's disease; burns; iatrogenic.

Clinical features

- Weakness
- ECG changes:
  - Peaked T waves, broad QRS, prolonged PR interval, loss of P waves, sinusoidal ECG pattern, VT/VF

Management

- K^+ 5.5–6.5 with no ECG changes: Stop/treat cause, consider exchange resin (e.g. calcium gluconate 15 g QDS [10 hours for effect], or furosemide IV for more rapid effect)
- K^+ greater than 6.5 or ECG changes:
  - 10 mL 10% Ca^{2+} gluconate over 15 min to stabilize myocardium (does not reduce serum K^+).
  - Soluble insulin 10 units (to increase cellular K^+ uptake) with +50 mL 50% glucose (to prevent hypoglycaemia) over 30 minutes.
  - Salbutamol nebulizers also increase cellular uptake.
- Failure of medical management may necessitate renal dialysis.

Hypokalaemia

Causes

- Fluid loss (diarrhoea, vomiting, diuretics); hyperaldosteronism; RTA (type 1+2); salbutamol/insulin (increased cellular uptake)

Clinical features

- Weakness
- ECG changes: ST depression, flattened T waves, U waves, broad QRS

Management

- K^+ >2.5 mmol/L: Oral K^+ replacement (e.g. Sando K 2 tabs TDS for 3/7); IV replacement if already on fluids or unable to take oral medication.

- K$^+$ <2.5 mmol/L: IV K$^+$ replacement – 20–40 mmol in 1 L fluid
  - Maximum rate of administration 10 mmol/h at a concentration less than 40 mmol/L.
- Faster rates and higher concentration are possible through central line with cardiac monitoring.

Sodium

Causes and management of significant derangements in sodium can be complex. Plasma concentrations must not be normalized rapidly (see below). Consider senior input.

Hypernatraemia (Na$^+$ >150 mmol/L)
Causes
- Fluid loss (diarrhoea, vomiting, diuretics); diabetes insipidus; salt overload (Cushing's syndrome, hyperaldosteronism, iatrogenic).

Clinical features
- Nausea/vomiting; confusion; convulsions, coma.

Management
- If euvolaemic/hypervolaemic: slow infusion of 5% glucose.
- If hypovolaemic: slow volume replacement with 0.9% NaCl.

Hyponatraemia (Na$^+$ <130 mmol/L)
- Fluid volume status, urine Na$^+$ and osmolarity also required for diagnosis.
- Follow local protocols or seek expert advice.

Causes
- Renal water loss (diuretics, Addison's disease, RTA); fluid loss (diarrhoea, vomiting); CCF, renal failure/nephotic syndrome, cirrhosis; SIADH.

Clinical features
- Nausea; confusion, convulsions, coma; muscle cramps, myoclonus.

Management
- If hypovolaemic: slow 0.9% saline infusion as there is a total body Na$^+$ deficit (hypertonic [1.8%, 3%] saline rarely used for rapid correction – do not use routinely as rapid correction of hyponatraemia may lead to central pontine myelinolysis) (max. daily change in serum Na$^+$ 8 mmol/L or 0.5 mmol/L/h).
- If euvolaemic/hypervolaemic: fluid restriction (e.g. 1.5 L/24h); Demeclocycline occasionally used in SIADH (causes an element of dehydration).

Calcium
Hypercalcaemia (Ca²⁺ >2.65 mmol/L)

Causes
- Hyperparathyroidism including ectopic secretion; bone metastases; hyperthyroidism, thiazide diuretics, milk-alkali syndrome (excess calcium intake).

Clinical features
- Cognitive/psychiatric disturbance, renal calculi, abdominal pain, constipation.
- ECG changes: shortened QT/PR interval.

Management
- First line:
    - Hydration, slow 0.9% saline infusion to encourage diuresis.
    - Furosemide may also be considered post-hydration.
- Second line: IV bisphosphonates used in severe hypercalcaemia (symptomatic, ECG changes, Ca^{2+} >3.0 mmol/L): 15–90 mg pamidronate, depending on Ca^{2+} level (zolendronate also used); 24 hours for effect; max effect at around 5 days.

Hypocalcaemia (Ca²⁺ <2.2 mmol/L)
Causes
- Vitamin D deficiency; hypoparathyroidism; hypomagnesaemia; hyperphosphataemia.

Clinical features
- Tetany; cognitive disturbance; convulsions, Chvostek's/Trousseau's sign.
- ECG changes: prolonged QT interval.

Management
- Replacement required if symptomatic, ECG changes or Ca^{2+}<2.0 mmol/L:
    - 10 mL 10% calcium gluconate/chloride IV slowly.

Magnesium
Hypomagnesaemia (Mg²⁺ <0.7 mmol/L)
Causes
- Diarrhoea, malabsorption; diuretics; acute tubular necrosis.

Clinical features
- Similar to hypocalcaemia; may also cause low K^+/Ca^{2+}, prolonged QT interval.

Management

- Mg^{2+} >0.5 mmol/L: Oral replacement usually adequate (unless symptomatic) – magnesium glycerophosphate 1–2 tabs TDS (unlicensed).
- Mg^{2+} <0.5 mmol/L:
  - IV replacement – 20 mmol $MgSO_4$ in 500 mL 0.9% saline over 12 h.
- If severe or life threatening features (seizures/arrhythmias) give 8 mmol $MgSO_4$ in 100 mL 0.9% saline over 15 minutes.

Phosphate

Hypophosphataemia (PO_4^{3-} <0.8 mmol/L)

Causes

- Decreased intake/absorption; vitamin D deficiency; hyperparathyroidism; diuretics; liver disease/alcohol; respiratory alkalosis; re-feeding syndrome.

Clinical features

- Myopathy/rhabdomyolysis, cardiomyopathy, acidosis, CNS disturbance (confusion, seizure, coma), respiratory failure.

Management

- PO_4^{3-} >0.4 mmol/L: Oral replacement usually adequate (improved dietary intake will help) – phosphate Sandoz 2 tabs TDS.
- PO_4^{3-} <0.4 mmol/L:
  - Requires IV replacement with Polyfusor® run at 9 mmol over 12 h (3.75 mL/h of PO_4^{3-} 100 mmol in 500 mL saline, or 7.5 mL/h of PO_4^{3-} 50 mmol in 500 mL saline).
  - May be infused at higher rate in critical care environment.
- PO_4^{3-} should be checked every 12 h.

16 Prescribing in diabetes

16.1 INSULIN AND PRESCRIBING IN DIABETES

PHARMACODYNAMICS

- Insulin is an endogenous peptide hormone produced by the beta cells of the islet of Langerhans in the endocrine pancreas.
- It acts to control serum glucose levels – daily output in health is equivalent to around 50 units.
- Insulin acts by binding to specific receptors on the extracellular surface of tissues including liver, fat, muscle and brain, which by several mechanisms results in a lowering of serum glucose by several mechanisms:
  - Uptake of glucose into cells (Fig. 16.1):
    - The insulin receptor has two subunits, the ß subunit contains a tyrosine kinase.
    - Binding of insulin to the extracellular receptor domain activates tyrosine kinase phosphorylation.
    - This induces intracellular insulin receptor substrate (IRS) to bind to the receptor, activating an intracellular protein cascade resulting in the translocation of GLUT-4 receptors to the cellular membrane and subsequent influx of glucose into the cell (see MICRO-print and Fig. 16.1).
  - Glycogen synthesis.
  - Increased protein synthesis.
  - Reduced hepatic glucose production.

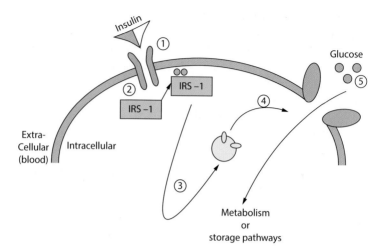

Fig. 16.1 Insulin-mediated uptake of glucose into cells via GLUT 4 channels. (1) Insulin binding to specific receptor; (2) recruitment and activation by phosphorylation of IRS-1; (3) IRS-1 activated protein cascade, (4) GLUT 4 transportation to cell membrane and exocytosis onto surface; (5) intracellular transport of glucose.

MICRO-print

Insulin glucose transporters

- Glucose is transported intracellularly via a number of specific transporters (GLUT). Only GLUT 4 receptors are activated by insulin.
  - GLUT 1: Fetal tissues and blood-brain barrier
  - GLUT 2: Bidirectional transporter found in a number of organs including the liver and pancreas (where it allows monitoring of glucose concentration and insulin release).
  - GLUT 3: Neurones.
  - GLUT 4: Striated muscle and fat tissues.

TYPES OF INSULIN

- Insulin has a half-life of only a few minutes once in the plasma, so the differing speeds of onset and lengths of action of the different types of insulin are determined by their rate of absorption after subcutaneous administration.

Quick acting

- Rapid onset of action (≤30 min) and short half-life (2–8 h).
- Administered prior to meals as part of maintenance regime.
- Intravenous administration when rapid/tight control of blood glucose (BG) is required (for example, in DKA).

Short-acting soluble insulin
- Recombinant human or animal insulins.
- Used for maintenance and when intravenous administration required.
- Examples: **Actrapid®, Humulin S®, Hypurin porcine/bovine neutral®**.
  - S/C onset/administration: 30 min, administer 20–30 min before carbohydrate meal.
  - IV administration gives a more rapid onset of action.
  - Peak serum concentration 2–4 h, duration 6–8 h.

Rapid acting insulin analogues
- Recombinant insulins with structural alterations to change their pharmacokinetic properties (i.e. more rapid onset of action).
- This allows greater flexibility of dosing as they do not have to be given in advance of meals.
- Examples: **Insulin lispro (Humalog®), insulin aspart (Novorapid/Novolog®), insulin glulisine (Apidra®)**.
  - S/C onset/administration: 10–20 min, administer with meals or up to 15 min after carbohydrate meal.
  - Peak serum concentration 1–3 h, duration 2–5 h (results in fewer hypos).

Intermediate/long acting
- Longer delay in onset and longer duration to provide basal insulin level.

Isophane insulin
- Recombinant insulins complexed with protamine compounds to alter the rate of absorption and prolong duration of action (intermediate acting).
- Examples: **Insulatard®, Humulin I®, Hypurin bovine/porcine isophane®**.
  - S/C onset/administration: 1.5 h, administered once or twice daily.
  - Peak serum concentration 4–12 h, duration 10–16 h.

Long-acting insulin analogues (lente insulin)
- Recombinant insulins with change in structure to alter absorption and distribution.
- **Insulin glargine (Lantus®)**:
  - Change of electrochemical structure alters solubility at physiological pH.
  - After subcutaneous injection most of the product precipitates out as crystals and then slowly re-dissolves, producing continued insulin release into plasma.
  - S/C onset/administration: 2 h, administer once daily in the morning.
  - Peak serum concentration 6–8 h (steady state at 2–4 OD doses), duration 24 h.

Drugs and practical prescribing

- **Insulin detemir (Levemir®):**
  - Change in structure produces rapid absorption after subcutaneous administration and subsequent binding to serum albumin.
  - Slow dissociation from albumin produces steady continuous insulin release into plasma.
  - S/C onset/administration: 2 h, administer once or twice daily.
  - Peak serum concentration 6–8 h (steady state after 2–3 BD doses), duration 16–24 h (dose dependent).

Mixed insulins

- Mixed insulins contain short acting soluble insulin/insulin analogues and isophane insulin in a fixed ratio.
- They provide basal insulin as well as pre-meal requirements.
- The numbers after the product name indicate ratio of short acting to isophane insulin.
- For example, Novomix 30 contains 30% short acting insulin, 70% isophane insulin.
- Examples:
  - Pre-mixed insulin (soluble insulin/isophane): **Humulin M3®**, **Hypurin porcine 30/70 mix®**.
    - S/C onset/administration: 30 min, administer 15–20 min before meals.
    - Peak serum concentration initial peak at 2–4 h, second peak at 6-8 h, duration 10–16 h.
  - Biphasic insulin analogues (insulin analogue/isophane): **Novomix 30®**, **Humalog 25®**, **Humalog 50®**.
    - S/C onset/administration: 10–20 min, administer with meals or up to 15 min after.
    - Peak serum concentration: initial peak at 1–3 h, second peak at 6–8 h, duration 10–16 h.

INSULIN REGIMES

Type 1 diabetes

- Patients with type 1 diabetes always require insulin as there is no endogenous production.
- These patients require a constant background of insulin and basal insulin requirements should never be omitted.
- Daily insulin requirements are approximately 0.5–1 unit/kg/day.
- Several insulin regimes are possible:
  - Twice daily mixed insulin before breakfast and evening meal.
  - Multiple injections with short acting insulin before meals, plus once or twice daily administration of intermediate/long acting insulin.

- Patients can be trained to estimate required pre-meal insulin doses based on the carbohydrate content of the meal (known as DAFNE – dose adjustment for normal eating).

> ## MICRO-facts
>
> Insulin should *never* be omitted entirely in patients with type 1 diabetes as this can result in dangerously high blood glucose levels and diabetic ketoacidosis.

Type 2 diabetes

- Patients with type 2 diabetes usually have some residual endogenous insulin production, and may be maintained purely on diet alterations or oral hypoglycaemic agents (see Ch. 9, Section 9.1).
- In the absence of oral carbohydrate intake (for example, if nil by mouth pre-surgery), it may be possible to simply monitor BG in these patients and avoid giving basal insulin or sliding insulin scales (see below).
- Difficulty in controlling blood glucose levels or poor tolerance of oral agents may necessitate insulin use, for example:
  - Oral agents used during day, with bedtime administration of intermediate/long acting insulin (usually glargine).
  - Twice daily mixed insulin before breakfast and evening meal (plus metformin if not contraindicated).
  - Patients with T2DM with no residual insulin production may require a regime similar to that used in T1DM – short acting insulin before meals plus once/twice daily intermediate/long acting insulin.
- Insulin requirements are often much larger than those seen in type 1 diabetics due to insulin resistance.

INSULIN AND DOSE CHANGES

- For patients with inadequate glycaemic control dose changes may be required.
- Before changing the dose consider causes of poor control:
  - Diet.
  - Concordance with insulin regimen (including appropriateness of regimen).
  - Precipitating factors (e.g. hyperglycaemia and intercurrent infection).
- Most settings will have their own local protocols which should be followed, below is an example of a typical regimen.

High blood sugars

- If BG persistently >11 mmol/L, or >17 mmol for >24 h, an increase in insulin or oral hypoglycaemic dose is required.

- A dose increase of 10% is usually appropriate.
- If BG is greater than 17 mmol/L, an increase of 15–20% may be necessary.
- If BG is persistently raised at certain times of day, consideration should be paid to the timing and also the type of insulin currently prescribed (in particular the dose and pharmacokinetic profile). For example:
  - If BG increased before lunch only, increase the short acting proportion of breakfast insulin dose by the appropriate percentage (as discussed above).
  - If BG increased before breakfast, increase the bedtime dose of long acting insulin (will require BG check overnight to ensure hypoglycaemia doesn't develop).

Low blood sugars

- Hypoglycaemia (normally defined as a BG <4 mmol/L) requires prompt recognition and management.
- A reduction in insulin or oral hypoglycaemic doses is indicated if:
  - A patient is having regular hypoglycaemic episodes.
  - There is an episode of severe hypoglycaemia (defined as BG <3 mmol/L).
- Insulin doses should be reduced by 25% in patients with type 1 diabetes.
- Doses of insulin or oral agents should be reduced by 25–50% in patients with type 2 diabetes.
- Similarly to hyperglycaemia, consideration must be paid to the dose and duration of action of the insulin.
- Early involvement of the local diabetes services is often indicated if there is difficulty gaining adequate control. For example:
  - If the BG is low before evening meals, decrease lunchtime dose of short acting insulin/mixed insulin or morning dose of long acting insulin.

MICRO-facts

Hypoglycaemia in type 1 diabetics
- Following a hypoglycaemic episode, the next dose of insulin due should *not* be omitted in patients with type 1 diabetes.
- If further episodes of hypoglycaemia are of concern (e.g. patient nil by mouth), basal insulin should be supplemented with carbohydrate administration, for example using a sliding scale.

AVOIDING PRESCRIBING ERRORS

- A large proportion of drug prescribing and administration errors involve the use of insulin, leading to serious morbidity and mortality.

Drugs and practical prescribing

- Avoiding prescribing errors:
  - Always write 'units' in full, not 'U' or 'IU' – this may be misread as a zero and result in ten times the intended dose being given.
  - Write the correct name of the insulin in full including any numbers or letters after the brand name.
  - The method of administration should be included in the prescription (for example vial, pre-filled pen).
  - The patient's recent glucose control and insulin use as well as their expected carbohydrate intake (i.e. how well they are eating currently) should be taken into account. Patients familiar with dose adjustment may be encouraged to assess their own requirements.
- Avoiding administration errors:
  - Always use dedicated insulin syringes for administering doses, and ensure that syringes are calibrated in 1-unit increments to allow accurate dosing.
  - Insulin syringes should also be used for measuring insulin prior to preparation of intravenous infusions – pre-filled syringes should be used if available.

> **MICRO-reference**
> National Patient Safety Agency. Safer administration of insulin. June 16, 2010. Available at: http://www.nrls.npsa.nhs.uk/ alerts/?entryid45=74287 (accessed March 22, 2014)

INSULIN INFUSIONS AND SLIDING SCALES

- Local policies are usually available. Most work upon similar principles and example regimens are shown below.
- Insulin infusions are required in certain circumstances for optimisation of blood glucose control.
- There are two core regimens, dependent on the indication:
  - Fixed rate insulin:
    - Diabetic emergencies: diabetic ketoacidosis (DKA)/hypersomolar hyperglycaemic state (see below).
  - Sliding scale (variable rate insulin):
    - Persistent hyperglycaemia
    - Nil by mouth/vomiting
    - Tight glucose control required
      - Fluctuant BG, e.g. severe intercurrent illness (sepsis etc)
      - Acute coronary syndromes
    - Peri-operative period (see below)

Fixed rate insulin (diabetic emergencies)

- Fixed-rate insulin infusions are now used in placed of sliding scale regimens, as they lead to more rapid correction of hyperglycaemia and resolution of ketoacidosis (in DKA).

Diabetic ketoacidosis (DKA)

- This is a combination of:
  - Blood glucose >10 mmol/L
  - Blood ketones >3 mmol/L
  - Venous bicarbonate <15 mmol/L
- Management is based around three main principles:
  - Fluid replacement
    - Patients presenting in DKA usually have significant fluid deficits, often estimated at around 100 mL/kg.
    - Crystalloid is used for fluid resuscitation and ongoing replacement, usually 0.9% saline.
    - Potassium supplementation is required in the replacement fluid (see below).
    - The rate of fluid administration depends upon the haemodynamic status of the patient (including hypotension). However, the aim is to restore the circulating volume as quickly as possible. A common regimen is as follows:
      - 1L 0.9% saline over 1 h, followed by
      - 1L 0.9% saline over 2 h
      - 1L 0.9% saline over 2 h
      - 1L 0.9% saline over 4 h
      - 1L 0.9% saline over 4 h
      - 1L 0.9% saline over 6 h
    - Further fluid replacement will depend on clinical assessment of fluid status. More cautious fluid replacement in pregnant or elderly patients, or those with heart or renal failure.
    - Once the blood glucose drops below 14 mmol/L (see below), an infusion of 10% dextrose at a rate of 125 mL/h should be started in addition to 0.9% saline fluid replacement, to prevent hypoglycaemia.
  - Correction of hyperglycaemia
    - Prescribe 50 units of **human soluble insulin** (e.g. **Actrapid®**) in 50 mL 0.9% saline and administer at 0.1 units/kg/h.
    - Targets of insulin therapy are:
      - Reduction of blood ketones concentration by 0.5 mmol/L/h
      - Reduction in blood glucose by 3 mmol/L/h
      - Increase in venous bicarbonate by 3 mmol/L/h
      - If these targets are not being met, an increase in the rate if insulin administration is required, 0.1 units/kg/h increments.

- Correction of electrolyte abnormalities
  - Patients tend to have low total body potassium and will require replacement as fluid status and hyperglycaemia are corrected.
  - Potassium should be given in all bags of fluid (except the first bag) as follows:
    - Serum K^+ <3.5 mmol/L: 40 mmol KCL per litre
    - Serum K^+ 3.5–5.5 mmol/L: 20 mmol KCL per litre
    - Serum K^+ >5.5: nil
    - If serum K^+ remains <3.5 mmol/L despite replacement, high concentration potassium replacement is likely to be required (via central venous catheter).
- Monitoring and further management:
  - Blood glucose and blood ketones should be measured hourly. Venous bicarbonate and potassium should be measured at baseline, at 1 hour and then at 2-hourly intervals.
  - Resolution of DKA is achieved once blood ketones <0.3 mmol/L and venous bicarbonate >15 mmol/L.
  - Those with resolved DKA who are not eating and drinking will require a change to a sliding scale regimen.
  - See below regarding continuation of insulin therapy.

Hyperosmolar hyperglycaemic state (HHS)

- Represents a severe hyperglycaemic state without significant ketonaemia.
  - Can be overlapped with DKA – discuss with diabetes team.
- Main features are:
  - Hypovolaemia
  - Hyperglycaemia, usually blood glucose >30 mmol/L (without significant ketonaemia or acidosis)
  - Serum osmolality >320 mosml/L
- Main principle of management is fluid replacement. Insulin is not usually required, unless there is significant ketonaemia or the rate of decrease in blood glucose is very slow.
  - Administration of fluid will in itself cause the blood glucose concentration to fall (sodium will rise, but this is usually acceptable provided serum osmolality falling).
- Potassium replacement is as in DKA, although potassium requirements likely to be less.
- If insulin is required, use fixed-rate insulin infusion starting at 0.05 units/kg/h.
- Correction of hyperosmolar state and hyperglycaemia likely to take several days (unlike DKA).

Drugs and practical prescribing

Sliding scale regimens
General principles

- These will vary according to local protocol however similar principles apply:
  - Insulin administered at a variable rate dependent on blood glucose.
  - Fluids run alongside to 'feed' insulin into cannula.
    - Type 1 diabetics require continuous administration of insulin so glucose must be run alongside as an infusion.
    - Type 2 diabetics require blood glucose control. Local policies vary, however many centres advocate an infusion containing some glucose to run alongside the insulin infusion.
    - Total maintenance fluid administration should take into account volume run along with sliding scale and may be prescribed separately.
      - i.e. prescription may contain insulin as per sliding scale, dextrose at set rate, and additional crystalloid to make up total maintenance volume.

Prescribing

- **Insulin**
  - Prescribed as 50 units soluble insulin in 50 mL 0.9% saline and run via a syringe driver following one of the regimens shown in Table 16.1.

Table 16.1 **Example intravenous insulin infusion regimens using insulin 50 units in 50 mL normal saline via infusion pump***

INTRAVENOUS INSULIN PRESCRIPTION – Insulin (human soluble) 50 units in 50 mLs sodium chloride 0.9%					
Start with standard insulin regimen. Check meter BG hourly and adjust insulin infusion rate accordingly.					
BLOOD GLUCOSE (MMOL/L)	STANDARD INSULIN REGIMEN (UNITS/H)	REDUCED REGIMEN (UNITS/H)	AUGMENTED REGIMEN 1 (UNITS/H)	AUGMENTED REGIMEN 2 (UNITS/H)	ALTERED REGIMEN 3 (UNITS/H)
0–39	0	0	0	0	
4–6.9	0.5	0	1	1	
7–8.9	1	0.5	2	2	
9–10.9	2	1	3	4	
11–13.9	3	2	4	6	
14–19.9	4	3	6	8	
≥20	6	4	9	12	

Start, date, time and nurse's signature
Discontinued date, time and nurse's signature
Date, time, and doctor's signature and bleep No.
*Includes augmented regimens for those not controlled on standard regimen.

- **Glucose (Dextrose)** and fluids
  - In Type 1 diabetics a dextrose 10% solution is run alongside the insulin infusion at a rate of 50 mL/h (i.e. 500 mL bag of 10% dextrose over 10 h). Maintenance fluids should be prescribed in addition.
  - In Type 2 diabetics fluid administration varies according to local policy, however dextrose 5% or dextrose 4% with saline 0.18% run at patient appropriate maintenance rates are potential alternatives.
    - If the blood glucose concentration is initially greater than 15 mmol/L, use 0.9% saline and switch to dextrose once BG is less than 15 mmol/L.
    - Do not switch back to saline if BG increases unless BG is greater than 20 mmol/L; increase insulin infusion rate as per regimen.
    - Concurrent TPN/NG feeds negates background glucose requirements provided they supply a sufficient amount of carbohydrate.
- Electrolytes
  - Serum electrolytes must be checked at least daily (more frequently if appropriate).
  - Potassium should be added as required (insulin infusion will cause a drop in serum potassium). For example:
    - Serum K$^+$ >5 mmol/L: no potassium required.
    - Serum K$^+$ <5 mmol/L: 20 mmol KCl per 500 mL 10% dextrose.
      - If <3.5 consider additional treatment
  - If BG falls outside target range after two hours of starting the sliding scale, use of an alternative/augmented infusion regime is required (Table 16.1).
  - Those in renal failure may not require the addition of potassium, though levels should still be checked.

Hypoglycaemia

- Stop insulin infusion and administer 100 mL 10% dextrose stat.
- Then return to dextrose 50 mL/h and monitor BG every 30 min until BG >6 mmol/l.
- Insulin can then be restarted using a reduced augmented regimen.

MICRO-facts

- Infusions of insulin and glucose must be run via infusion pumps and through the same intravenous line.
- If insulin and glucose infusions are run through separate lines, occlusion of one line will produce severe hypoglycaemia or hyperglycaemia respectively.

Restarting patients usual insulin/oral hypoglycaemic regimen:
- When patients are eating and drinking normally (and not ketotic) it may be appropriate to stop the sliding scale and restart their normal medications.
- Normal medications should be restarted prior to stopping sliding scale to allow them time to have an effect and allow seamless therapy.
  - Subcutaneous insulin should be administered before the patient's meal and the insulin and dextrose infusions should be tailed off from at least 30 min to 1 h after administration of the subcutaneous dose (depending on local polices).
  - Exact protocol for oral medications varies dependent on type and mechanism of action.
    - Typically they should be also be administered at planned time (e.g. prior to meal) and sliding scale tailed off in the hours following this.
    - Ensure normal renal function (particularly for restarting metformin).
- Reduction of usual doses may be appropriate if the patient is not expected to eat as much as normal.

PRE-OPERATIVE PATIENTS

Use local policies if applicable; below outlines an example of procedure:
- Diabetic patients should be first on the morning list for surgery/procedures.
  - If the procedure is in the afternoon, a light breakfast and morning insulin/oral agents can be given (omit long acting insulins).
- Diabetic patients who are required not to eat prior to surgery or a procedure need their BG checked regularly, and may require an insulin infusion depending on the length of time they must fast:
  - Patients with type 1 diabetes will require an insulin infusion if they are expected to fast for more than a few hours (otherwise hourly BG monitoring is adequate).
  - Patients with type 2 diabetes who are expected to eat within 24 hours can have all insulin/oral agents omitted on the morning of the procedure and carefully monitored:
    - If BG rises >15 mmol/L, an insulin infusion is required.
    - Patients not expected to eat within 24 h also need an insulin infusion.
- In unwell patients with diabetes, blood glucose should be monitored regularly:
  - If BG <14 mmol/L and patient well: Continue to monitor.

- 14 mmol/L > BG <25 mmol/L and patient normally on insulin but well: Continue to monitor.
- If unwell with ketonuria (greater than 2+ on urine dip) or severe hyperglycaemia (BG >25 mmol/L), or vomiting/not eating: Start sliding scale.
- If unwell with ketonuria/BG> 25 mmol/L plus bicarbonate <17 mmol/L or serum osmolality >330 mOsm/L: Treat as DKA.

17 Immunosuppressants

17.1 IMMUNOSUPPRESSANT AND IMMUNOMODULATORY DRUGS

- Drugs that modulate the effects of the immune system are used in the treatment of autoimmune disease, as well as the prevention of rejection of transplanted organs. Some agents also have anti-cancer properties.
- These agents should only be used under specialist supervision (especially initiation), but as patients on immunomodulatory drugs are commonly encountered in everyday practice, it is important to be familiar with their use and properties.

AZATHIOPRINE AND 6-MERCAPTOPURINE (6-MP)

Pharmacodynamics

- Active metabolites act as structural purine analogues, inhibiting de novo purine synthesis:
    - Inhibition of purine synthesis impairs DNA synthesis and cell proliferation, especially in cells that are rapidly dividing (e.g. lymphocytes).
    - Impairment of lymphocyte proliferation and function results in immunosuppression and they can therefore act as cytotoxic agents.
- **Azathioprine** is a prodrug of 6-MP; both are metabolized to active metabolites (mainly 6-thioguanine) with immunosuppressive effects.

Pharmacokinetics

- Metabolism: Metabolism is via several pathways involving multiple enzymes including thiopurine methyltransferase (TPMT). Differing polymorphisms of TPMT exist making some individuals poor metabolizers and at risk of toxicity (see below).
- Elimination: Xanthine oxidase involved in degradation to elimination products – inhibitors of this enzyme (e.g. allopurinol) reduce elimination with significant toxicity risks.

Indications

- Prevention of solid organ rejection.
- Immunosuppression in autoimmune conditions (e.g. rheumatoid arthritis, inflammatory bowel disease).

Cautions

- Pregnancy.
- Active intestinal disease.

Contraindications

- Absent TPMT activity (high risk of marrow suppression).

Adverse effects

- Marrow suppression: More common in individuals with low TPMT activity (resulting in accumulation of toxic metabolites).
- Hypersensitivity reactions.
- Hepatotoxicity: Including cholestasis and hepatitis.
- Pancreatitis: Azathioprine.

Important interactions

- See pharmacokinetics above.

Special requirements

- TPMT activity should be measured before starting treatment.
- Frequent monitoring of blood counts is necessary.
- The bioavailability of different preparations varies, and formulations should not be changed without specialist advice.

METHOTREXATE

Pharmacodynamics

- Two main mechanisms of action:
  - Anti-cancer (high-dose): competitively inhibits the action of dihydrofolate reductase (DHFR):
    - DHFR catalyzes formation of active folic acid metabolites required for purine and DNA synthesis (and thus methotrexate impairs DNA and RNA synthesis).
    - Rapidly dividing cells predominantly affected by inhibition of purine synthesis.
    - Purine synthesis may be restored by administration of folic acid or folinic acid (see MICRO-print box).
  - Anti-inflammatory (low-dose): Inhibition of enzymes involved in purine metabolism leads to inhibition of macrophage and lymphocyte function.

Pharmacokinetics

- Good oral bioavailability. Administered parenterally or intrathecally as cancer chemotherapy. Mainly renal elimination.

Indications

- Rheumatoid arthritis (and other rheumatological inflammatory conditions).
- Inflammatory bowel disease.
- Psoriasis.
- Malignant disease (high-dose).

Cautions

- Hepatic disease.
- Blood disorders.
- Significant effusions/fluid collections (drug may accumulate).

Contraindications

- Active infection or immunodeficiency.
- Pregnancy (contraception required for 3 months following cessation of treatment).

Adverse effects

- Marrow suppression: Onset can be rapid; increased risk if concomitant use of other drugs with anti-folate activity (e.g. trimethoprim and sulfamethoxazole [both independently and as co-trimoxazole]).
- Mucositis: Oral or gastrointestinal ulceration, risk reduced by folate supplementation (see MICRO-print box).
- Pneumonitis: Especially in rheumatoid arthritis.
- Hepatotoxicity.
- Skin disorders: Including photosensitivity, TEN and SJS.

Important interactions

- Other less commonly encountered interactions exist – see other interactions source.
- NSAIDs (including aspirin): Reduced methotrexate excretion.
- Penicillin: Methotrexate toxicity due to reduced excretion.
- Anti-folates: See above; phenytoin also increases antifolate effects.

Special requirements

- Monitoring of blood counts, renal and hepatic function is required before and during therapy and patients should be advised to report any symptoms of infection.
- For inflammatory conditions, methotrexate is administered as a single weekly dose – patients should be educated about their dose, how often and on which day it is taken.
- Daily administration of methotrexate in non-cancer patients is a 'never' event – i.e. it should never happen.

> **MICRO-print**
> **Folate supplementation in methotrexate therapy**
>
> - **Folic acid** may be administered to patients who are receiving methotrexate to reduce the risk of mucositis and myelosuppression.
>   - It is often given as 5 mg weekly (more frequent if required), but should not be administered on the same day as methotrexate.
> - **Folinic acid** is used as rescue therapy in mocusitis or myelosuppression due to methotrexate (usually in the context of high-dose cancer chemotherapy or overdose).
>   - Folinic acid is readily converted to usable folate derivatives without the action of dihydrofolate reductase – therefore it allows DNA and RNA synthesis to continue even when dihydrofolate reductase is inhibited by methotrexate.

SULFASALAZINE

- See Ch. 7, Section 7.2.

LEFLUNOMIDE ARAVA®

Pharmacodynamics

- Pyrimidine synthesis inhibitor.
- Active metabolite inhibits dihydroorotate dehydrogenase involved in pyrimidine synthesis.
- Leads to reduced T cell proliferation and B cell antibody production.

Pharmacokinetics

- Long $t_{1/2}$ means loading doses required.
- Washout (total body drug clearance) of active metabolites may be required in toxicity, when changing drugs or prior to conception.
- Cholestyramine or activated charcoal used.

Indications

- Severe rheumatoid arthritis.
- Psoriatic arthritis.

Cautions

- Blood disorders; recent treatment with other immunosuppressant agents.
- History of tuberculosis.

Contraindications

- Pregnancy (contraception required for 3 months following cessation of treatment).

Adverse effects

- GI disturbance (including mucosal ulceration).
- Hepatotoxicity: May be severe.
- Marrow suppression (rare).

Important interactions

- Increased risk of toxicity when administered with **methotrexate**.

Special requirements

- Monitor hepatic function regularly during treatment.

CICLOSPORIN

Pharmacodynamics

- Immunosuppression as a result of binding to T cell proteins and action as a calcineurin inhibitor.
- Calcineurin normally activates IL-2 (interleukin 2) transcription; inhibition prevents IL-2 release and subsequent T cell activation.
- Unlike most immunosuppressive agents, ciclosporine does not cause marrow suppression.

Pharmacokinetics

- Poor oral bioavailability. Metabolized by hepatic CYP450 enzymes.

Indications

- Prevention of solid organ rejection/bone marrow graft rejection.
- Severe ulcerative colitis.
- Rheumatoid arthritis.
- Atopic dermatitis, psoriasis.

Cautions

- Renal impairment.
- Hypertension (discontinue if uncontrollable).
- Avoid excessive UV exposure.

Contraindications

- Uncontrolled infection and malignancy.

Adverse effects

- Nephrotoxicity: Significant risk, changes in renal parenchyma may occur over time.
- Electrolyte/metabolic disturbance: Hyperuricaemia, hyperkalaemia, hypomagnesaemia, hyperlipidaemia, hypercholesterolaemia.
- Hepatotoxicity.

Important interactions

- Grapefruit juice significantly increases serum concentrations.

- Serum levels likely to be affected by inhibitors or inducers of hepatic CYP450 enzymes.
- Multiple interactions – see other interactions source.
- Concomitant administration with tacrolimus contraindicated (except in transplant patients) due to risk of ciclosporin toxicity.

Special requirements

- Monitor renal function, hepatic function and electrolytes.
- Dose adjusted according to serum ciclosporin concentration.

ANTI-TNF-α AGENTS

Pharmacodynamics

- These agents bind to tumour necrosis factor-alpha (TNF-α) and prevent its interaction with macrophage and T cell surface receptors.
- Inhibition of macrophages and T cells prevents inflammatory processes.
- Most are monoclonal antibodies (mAb) except **Etanercept** which is a 'fusion protein' (a soluble TNF receptor protein fused with an antibody constant region, as opposed to complete antibody).

Pharmacokinetics

- Require parenteral administration (IV or subcutaneous).
- Long $t_{1/2}$ means weekly (or even monthly) administration is possible.

Indications

- Rheumatoid arthritis (after failure of DMARD therapy).
- Used in conjunction with methotrexate (or as monotherapy if not tolerated).
- Inflammatory bowel disease.
- Psoriasis.

Cautions

- Latent tuberculosis.
- Demyelination (may exacerbate disease, including multiple sclerosis).
- Malignancy (or history of malignancy).

Contraindications

- Severe infections.
- Significant heart failure.

Adverse effects

- Infection: Especially activation of latent tuberculosis (also bacterial infections, hepatitis B reactivation).
- Blood disorders: Anaemia, thrombocytopaenia, leucopaenia etc.
- Hypersensitivity reactions.
- Autoantibody formation: Rarely may cause SLE-like illness.

Examples

- **Infliximab (Remicade®):** Mouse-human chimeric mAb
- **Adalimumab (Humira®):** Human mAb
- **Golimumab (Simponi®):** Human mAb
- **Certolizomab pegol (Cimzia®):** PEGylated FAB' fragment of humanized mAb
- **Etanercept (Enbrel®):** TNF fusion protein (see above)

Special requirements

- Patients should be investigated for latent tuberculosis prior to treatment (Mantoux test is initial investigation).
- Anti-TNF therapy can begin two months after start of treatment of active TB; prophylactic treatment can be given concurrently.

MICRO-print

Cytokine modulators and monoclonal antibodies

There are an ever-increasing number of cytokine modulating drugs available for the treatment of conditions with an immunological basis. (See Table 7.1)

Table 17.1 **Cytokine modulators**

CYTOKINE MODULATOR	MECHANISM (TARGET CYTOKINE/RECEPTOR)	INDICATION
Anakinra	IL-2 receptor	Rheumatoid arthritis
Rituximab	CD-20	Lymphoma, autoimmune disease
Tocilizumab	IL-6 receptor	Autoimmune disease, myeloma, prostate cancer
Belimumab	B-cell activating factor	Autoimmune disease
Basiliximab	IL-2 receptor	Prevention of renal transplant rejection
Belatacept	Acts as fusion protein preventing T cell costimulation	Prevention of renal transplant rejection
Ofatumumab	CD-20	Chronic lymphocytic leukaemia
Natalizumab	α4-integrin	Relapsing-remitting multiple sclerosis
Abatacept	Acts as fusion protein preventing T cell costimulation	Rheumatoid arthritis

Drugs and practical prescribing

MICRO-print

Other immunosuppressant agents

Cyclophosphamide

- Potent immunosuppressant, also used as cancer chemotherapy. Alkylation of cell DNA leads to cell death (especially proliferating lymphoid cells).
- Adverse effects:
  - *Marrow suppression:* Especially at high doses (mainly used in cancer chemotherapy).
  - *Haemorrhagic cystitis:* Due to production of a toxic urinary metabolite – prevention possible by administration of **Mesna (Uromitexan®)**.
  - Cardiotoxicity.

Mycophenolate mofetil

- Active metabolite inhibits B and T cell responses; used in prevention of solid organ and stem cell transplant rejection, and increasingly in autoimmune disease (rheumatoid arthritis, SLE etc.).
- Most important adverse effect is marrow suppression.

Tacrolimus

- Acts as calcineurin inhibitor (see *ciclosporin*), preventing T cell IL-2 production
- Used in prevention of renal transplant rejection, as well as in some autoimmune conditions and topically in severe eczema.
- Main adverse effects are nephrotoxicity and electrolyte disturbances (see ciclosporin).

Sirolimus

- Binds to T cell proteins and prevents activation by IL-2 and other inflammatory cytokines.
- Used in prevention of renal transplant rejection.
- Commonly causes marrow suppression.

18 Inotropes

18.1 INOTROPIC DRUGS (REFERENCE ONLY)

BACKGROUND

This chapter is included to aid understanding of adrenoceptors and their physiological relevance to clinical practice.

- Numerous agents are used for their interactions with the autonomic nervous system and the augmentation of cardiovascular function that this allows.
- Adequate cardiovascular function is a product of several variables:
  - Cardiac output (CO) = heart rate × stroke volume (contractility).
  - Systemic blood pressure (SBP) = cardiac output × systemic vascular resistance (SVR).
- The agents discussed below may provide cardiovascular support where compromise of any of these variables results in haemodynamic instability. Several physiological mechanisms may be exploited at once (most agents act on multiple receptors):
  - Inotropes: increase the contractility of the heart (positive inotropy) via stimulation of cardiac adrenoceptors. Increase cardiac output.
  - Chronotropes: increase heart rate due to cardiac adrenoceptor agonism, increasing cardiac output.
  - Vasopressors: stimulate adrenoceptors in the peripheral vasculature, causing smooth muscle contraction. This increases systemic vascular resistance to maintain blood pressure and an adequate organ perfusion pressure.
- Due to the potent effects of these agents and the need for careful monitoring of cardiovascular parameters, their use is limited to areas where such monitoring is available (e.g. critical care or operating theatres).

Drugs and practical prescribing

Table 18.1 Drug list (for reference only)

CLASS	AGENT	RECEPTOR AFFINITY	ACTION	INDICATIONS	ADVERSE EFFECTS
Sympathomimetics	Adrenaline	Non-specific adrenoceptor agonist α_1, α_2; β_1, β_2	Inotrope, chronotrope; vasopressor (vasodilatation at low doses)	Cardiopulmonary resuscitation; hypotension (especially post-resuscitation); anaphylaxis	Hypertension, arrhythmias, dyspnoea, pulmonary oedema, hyperglycaemia, peripheral ischaemia, tissue necrosis
	Noradrenaline	α_1, α_2; $\beta_1 >> \beta_2$	Vasopressor; inotrope	Hypotension (especially in sepsis)	Peripheral ischaemia; hypertension; headache; confusion, psychosis; dyspnoea; urinary retention
	Metaraminol	Mainly α_1, some β receptor activity	Vasopressor	Hypotension (especially related to anaesthesia)	
	Phenylephrine	α_1 (β receptor activity at high doses)	Vasopressor	Hypotension (especially related to anaesthesia)	
	Dopamine	D_1, $D_2 > \beta > \alpha$ (dose dependant)	Vasopressor; inotrope at higher doses	Cardiogenic shock	Chest pain, palpitations, dyspnoea, headache

(Continued)

Table 18.1 (*Continued*) **Drug list (for reference only)**

CLASS	AGENT	RECEPTOR AFFINITY	ACTION	INDICATIONS	ADVERSE EFFECTS
	Dobutamine	$\beta_1 > \beta_2 >>> \alpha$	Inotrope	Cardiogenic shock	Hypo/hypertension, arrhythmias, dyspnoea, fever, eosinophilia
	Dopexamine	$\beta_2 > \beta_1 >>> \alpha$	Inotrope	Severe heart failure	Arrhythmias, angina, myocardial infarction, dyspnoea
	Isoprenaline	$\beta_2, \beta_1 >>> \alpha$	Chronotrope, inotrope	Bradycardia; AV nodal block	Arrhythmias, pulmonary oedema, dyspnoea, anxiety, blurred vision
Phosphodiesterase-3 inhibitors	Milrinone	PDE-3 inhibition increases cAMP	Inotrope; vasodilator	Severe heart failure	Ventricular ectopics; arrhythmias including ventricular tachycardia; hypotension
Calcium sensitisers	Levosimendan	Increased sensitivity to calcium increases myocyte contractility	Inotrope	Severe decompensated heart failure (expensive)	Arrhythmias, hypokalaemia, myocardial infarction

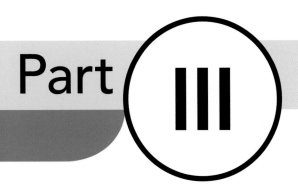

Part III

Self-assessment

19 Adverse drug reactions

CASE PRESENTATION 1

A 47-year-old man with previously normal renal function has just started taking lisinopril for hypertension.

Question 1

Which of the following is the *most likely* adverse effect to be caused by lisinopril?

ADVERSE EFFECT OPTIONS

A. Acute renal failure
B. Angioedema
C. Dry cough
D. Hepatitis
E. Hypokalaemia

CASE PRESENTATION 2

A 22-year-old woman who is being treated for pyelonephritis in hospital develops severe muscle spasms and increased tone in her left hand and arm. You suspect a dystonic reaction.

Question 2

Which of the following drugs is *most likely* to have caused this adverse reaction.

ADVERSE EFFECT OPTIONS

A. Cyclizine
B. Gentamicin
C. Ibuprofen
D. Metoclopramide
E. Morphine

CASE PRESENTATION 3

A 36-year-old man is undergoing treatment for tuberculosis. During the continuation phase of treatment he is diagnosed with a DVT and started on warfarin. After three months he completes his TB treatment. A few weeks later he presents with heavy epistaxis. His INR is 11.0.

Question 3

Interaction between warfarin and which of the following drugs is *most likely* to have resulted in this adverse effect?

ADVERSE EFFECT OPTIONS

A. Ethambutol
B. Isoniazid
C. Pyrazinamide
D. Pyridoxine (vitamin B6)
E. Rifampicin

CASE PRESENTATION 4

A 65-year-old diabetic man is taking metformin and gliclazide at maximum doses. He has recently had a viral illness and not been eating. He presents to the Emergency Department (ED) with a blood glucose of 1.6 mmol/L. His GCS is 6/15.

Question 4

Which of the following is the *most appropriate* initial management of this adverse drug reaction?

ADVERSE EFFECT OPTIONS

A. 1L 0.9% saline over 1 h
B. 1 mg glucagon IM
C. 50 mL 50% glucose IV
D. 100 mL sugary soft drink (e.g. Lucozade®)
E. 10 units quick-acting insulin

CASE PRESENTATION 5

A 71-year-old woman with osteoarthritis and hypertension presents to the ED with sudden onset haematemesis and abdominal pain.

Question 5

Which of the following drugs is *most likely* to have caused this adverse drug reaction?

ADVERSE EFFECT OPTIONS

A. Amlodipine
B. Bendroflumethiazide
C. Diclofenac
D. Paracetamol
E. Simvastatin

CASE PRESENTATION 6

A 56-year-old man is being treated for a *Pseudomonas* spp. wound infection with piperacillin/tazobactam and gentamicin.

Question 6

Which of the following is the *most likely* adverse drug reaction to be caused by gentamicin?

ADVERSE EFFECT OPTIONS

A. Cholestasis
B. Neuromuscular weakness
C. Rash
D. Renal impairment
E. Visual loss

CASE PRESENTATION 7

A 65-year-old man with known hypertensive heart failure presents to the ED with left ventricular failure and rapid atrial fibrillation. He is given intravenous verapamil to control his ventricular rate. He quickly develops complete heart block and requires emergency transvenous pacing.

Question 7

Interaction between verapamil and which of the following drugs is *most likely* to have resulted in this adverse effect?

ADVERSE EFFECT OPTIONS

A. Aspirin
B. Bisoprolol
C. Furosemide
D. Ramipril
E. Spironolactone

CASE PRESENTATION 8

A 70-year-old woman is taking warfarin for paroxysmal atrial fibrillation.
She has been confused for several days due to a urinary tract infection.
Her INR is 9.4. She presents with sudden onset left-sided weakness and
a fixed dilated right pupil, which a CT shows to be due to an intra-cerebral
bleed.

Question 8

Which of the following is the *most appropriate* initial management of this
adverse drug reaction?

ADVERSE EFFECT OPTIONS

A. 10 mg vitamin K IV
B. 40 mg dalteparin subcutaneously
C. 2 units fresh-frozen plasma (FFP)
D. 500 IU prothrombin complex concentrate (Beriplex®)
E. 1 g tranexamic acid IV

ANSWERS

Answer 1: C

(See Ch. 5, Section 5.5)

- A: Acute renal failure may complicate ACE inhibitor use, but is unlikely in someone without pre-existing renal or renovascular disease.
- B: Angioedema is a serious but infrequent adverse effect associated with ACE inhibitors such as lisinopril.
- C: Persistent dry cough is commonly associated with ACE inhibitors, and commonly necessitates discontinuation of the drug.
- D: Hepatitis is a rare adverse effect associated with ACE inhibitors.
- E: ACE inhibitors typically cause hyperkalaemia, not hypokalaemia.

Answer 2: D

(See Ch. 7, Section 7.4)

- A: Cyclizine rarely causes dystonic reactions.
- B: Does not cause dystonic reactions.
- C: Does not cause dystonic reactions.
- D: Metoclopramide is an anti-emetic that is associated with extrapyramidal adverse effects and dystonic reactions, especially when administered to young women.
- E: Does not cause dystonic reactions.

Answer 3: E

- A: No significant interactions with warfarin. Also not used in continuation phase of TB treatment.
- B: No significant interactions with warfarin.
- C: No significant interactions with warfarin. Also not used in continuation phase of TB treatment.
- D: No significant interactions with warfarin.
- E: Rifampicin is a potent liver enzyme inducer and will increase metabolism of warfarin when given concurrently. When rifampicin is discontinued, if warfarin is continued at the same dose the INR will quickly become supra-therapeutic. This may result in excessive or spontaneous bleeding.

Answer 4: C

- A: The patient may be dehydrated and require intravenous fluid replacement, but this is not the first priority.
- B: Glucagon is effective at raising the blood glucose, but is usually used when IV administration of drugs/fluids is not possible.
- C: This is the quickest and most effective way of raising the blood glucose, particularly in a patient with reduced consciousness.
- D: This should be avoided in a patient with reduced consciousness, as there is a high risk of aspiration. This would be appropriate initial management in a patient with full consciousness who is able to swallow.
- E: This patient needs glucose administration, not insulin! This will decrease the blood glucose further.

Answer 5: C

(See Ch. 10, Section 10.3)

- A: Calcium channel antagonists are not associated with GI bleeding.
- B: Thiazide diuretics may cause gastrointestinal disturbances but are not associated with GI bleeding.
- C: All NSAIDs are associated with gastrointestinal irritation and bleeding, and are a significant cause of drug-related morbidity and mortality. Long-term use should be avoided if possible, especially in the elderly. Gastric protection with a proton-pump inhibitor may be indicated to reduce the risk of gastrointestinal bleeding.
- D: Paracetamol does not cause significant gastro-intestinal disturbance and is rarely associated with GI bleeding.
- E: Statins may very rarely cause gastric irritation but are not associated with significant GI bleeding.

Self-assessment

Answer 6: D

- A: Gentamicin does not cause cholestasis.
- B: Gentamicin may very rarely cause neuromuscular weakness when given in very high doses.
- C: Rash does occur rarely with gentamicin use, but is much more commonly due to beta-lactam antibiotics.
- D: Aminoglycosides are nephrotoxic and may quickly cause renal impairment, especially at high serum concentrations or when used concurrently with other nephrotoxic drugs.
- E: Aminoglycosides are ototoxic at high serum levels; they do not cause visual loss.

Answer 7: B

(See Ch. 5, Section 5.6)

- A: No significant interaction with verapamil.
- B: This patient is likely to be taking a beta-receptor antagonist. Verapamil (and other non-dihydropyrimidine calcium channel antagonists) should not normally be co-administered with beta antagonists as both drugs produce AV nodal blockade. Concurrent use may result in high grade AV block and a significant reduction in cardiac contractility.
- C: Additive antihypertensive action, but unlikely to result in heart block.
- D: Additive antihypertensive action, but unlikely to result in heart block.
- E: Additive antihypertensive action, but unlikely to result in heart block.

Answer 8: D

(See Ch. 5, Section 5.10)

- A: Vitamin K is effective at reversing the effects of warfarin anticoagulation, but takes 6–8 hours to have an effect, so is not appropriate for immediate reversal of coagulopathy in emergency situations.
- B: Dalteparin is an anticoagulant and so will exacerbate any bleeding.
- C: FFP contains clotting factors present in human plasma, but is insufficient to rapidly reverse anticoagulation in severe or life-threatening bleeding.
- D: Prothrombin complex concentrate contains all the vitamin K-dependent clotting factors (II, VII, IX, X, protein C and S) and is able to rapidly reverse life-threatening bleeding due to warfarin anticoagulation. It is very expensive and is only prescribed after discussion with a senior haematologist.
- E: Tranexamic acid is an anti-fibrinolytic and is effective at reducing bleeding by preventing clot breakdown, especially in trauma. It is not suitable for the treatment of bleeding associated with warfarin associated anticoagulation.

Communicating information

CASE PRESENTATION 1

A 76-year-old woman attends her GP with a history of intermittent palpitations. An ECG during an attack reveals atrial fibrillation. She has a history of hypertension and had a TIA one year previously. She is advised to start warfarin to reduce her risk of stroke, to which she agrees.

Question 1

Select the *most appropriate* information item to communicate to the patient.

INFORMATION OPTIONS

A. Alcohol consumption is contraindicated.
B. Blood tests are not required after the first month.
C. Excessive bleeding is the most important adverse effect.
D. The different-coloured tablets are interchangeable.
E. Warfarin may cause hypotension and dizziness.

CASE PRESENTATION 2

A 14-year-old female patient presents with polyuria, polydipsia, weight loss and marked glycosuria. After further investigations, a diagnosis of type 1 diabetes is made and she is started on an insulin regime composed of mealtime short-acting insulin and bedtime insulin glargine.

Question 2

Select the *most appropriate* information item to communicate to the patient.

INFORMATION OPTIONS

A. Insulin doses should be omitted during times of illness when the patient is not eating.
B. Insulin treatment is likely to be temporary.
C. Mealtime insulin doses should be administered just after meals.
D. Subcutaneous insulin injections should always be made at the same site to avoid excessive scarring.

E. Symptoms and signs of hypoglycaemia and the importance of readily available high-sugar foods to raise blood glucose.

CASE PRESENTATION 3

A 19-year-old woman was diagnosed with asthma 6 months ago. She is having frequent episodes of breathlessness and is using her salbutamol inhaler several times a week. You decide to add in a regular inhaled corticosteroid.

Question 3

Select the *most appropriate* information item to communicate to the patient.

INFORMATION OPTIONS

A. A salbutamol inhaler will no longer be required.
B. A spacer device reduces the amount of drug delivered to the lung.
C. Inhaled steroids should be taken during an asthma attack to relieve symptoms.
D. The patient should rinse the mouth with water after each administration.
E. Tremor is a common adverse effect of an ICS.

CASE PRESENTATION 4

A 56-year-old woman who has suffered with painful and swollen joints for 2 years is diagnosed with rheumatoid arthritis. She is to be started on methotrexate to prevent disease progression.

Question 4

● Select the *most appropriate* information item to communicate to the patient.

INFORMATION OPTIONS

A. Blood tests are required weekly during treatment.
B. Methotrexate should not be taken together with NSAID drugs (e.g. ibuprofen).
C. Methotrexate treatment for rheumatoid arthritis should be taken once-weekly.
D. Pneumonitis is a common adverse effect.
E. Sore throat and fever are common adverse effects that can be treated with simple analgesia.

CASE PRESENTATION 5

A 66-year-old man suffers from refractory paroxysmal atrial fibrillation which has failed to respond to beta-blockers. His cardiologist decides to start him on amiodarone to maintain his sinus rhythm.

Question 5

Select the *most appropriate* information item to communicate to the patient.

INFORMATION OPTIONS

A. An itchy rash is a common adverse effect related to duration of treatment.
B. Any visual disturbance is always irreversible.
C. Missed doses will result in a significant reduction in treatment efficacy.
D. New respiratory symptoms (cough, breathlessness etc.) should be reported immediately.
E. There are no significant drug-drug interactions related to amiodarone therapy.

CASE PRESENTATION 6

A 70-year-old woman has recently had a DEXA bone scan and was found to have a marked reduction in bone mineral density. She is started on risedronate to reduce her risk of pathological fractures.

Question 6

Select the *most appropriate* information item to communicate to the patient.

INFORMATION OPTIONS

A. Bisphosphonates are associated with an increased risk of stroke.
B. Osteonecrosis of the jaw is a common adverse effect of bisphosphonates.
C. Risedronate should be taken before bed.
D. Risedronate should be taken monthly for the treatment of osteoporosis.
E. Risedronate should be taken on an empty stomach and washed down with a glass of water.

ANSWERS

Answer 1: C

- A: Alcohol consumption can affect warfarin and the INR, but regular moderate intake should not cause significant fluctuations. Consumption of large volumes of alcohol (bingeing) is likely to result in alterations in warfarin metabolism and the INR and should be avoided.
- B: INR monitoring is required for the duration of treatment, although the frequency of monitoring will decrease once a stable INR is achieved.
- C: There is increased risk of bleeding, especially if the INR exceeds the target range. Any prolonged or serious bleeding should receive prompt medical attention.

- D: Warfarin tablets are colour-coded according to dose. Tablets should not be used interchangeably as this may result in a significant under- or overdose.
- E: Warfarin treatment is not associated with hypotension (in the absence of severe haemorrhage).

Answer 2: E

(See Ch. 16, Section 16.1)

- A: Omission of insulin should be avoided in those with type 1 diabetes due to risk of developing diabetic ketoacidosis. This is especially true during inter-current illness, which may precipitate DKA. Blood glucose levels should be monitored closely and dose adjustments made as required.
- B: Insulin therapy in type 1 diabetes is life-long.
- C: Mealtime doses of short-acting insulin should be administered about 20–30 minutes before mealtimes.
- D: Insulin injection sites should be rotated to minimize bruising and the risk of fat necrosis.
- E: The most important adverse effect of insulin therapy is hypoglycaemia, and patients should be aware of the signs and symptoms of low blood sugar and ways to correct it.

Answer 3: D

(See Ch. 6, Section 6.3)

- A: Although an ICS should reduce the frequency of exacerbation, the patient should still carry a salbutamol inhaler as 'reliever' therapy in case of an exacerbation.
- B: Spacer devices increase the amount of drug that reaches the small airways and also reduce drug deposition in the oropharynx.
- C: Inhaled corticosteroids are effective in reducing the frequency of asthma exacerbations. They are not effective treatment during an exacerbation.
- D: Drug deposition in the oropharynx can lead to oropharyngeal candidiasis and other local infections; the mouth should be rinsed with water after ICS administration to remove any deposited drug.
- E: Tremor is associated with beta 2 agonist use (e.g. salbutamol), not inhaled corticosteroids.

Answer 4: C

(See Ch. 17, Section 17.1)

- A: Blood count and liver function monitoring are required every few weeks during initiation of therapy; after which blood tests are required every 3 months.
- B: The co-administration of methotrexate and NSAIDs is effective in rheumatic disease, and may be used together with careful monitoring.

- C: When used for non-cancer indications, methotrexate is administered once-weekly. Patients should be counseled on the dangers of daily dosing.
- D: Pneumonitis is a rare complication of methotrexate therapy. It is however associated with methotrexate use in the treatment of rheumatoid arthritis.
- E: Patients should be warned about the possibility of bone marrow suppression and the importance of recognizing and reporting symptoms of potentially severe infections.

Answer 5: D

(See Ch. 5, Section 5.3)

- A: The most common adverse skin reaction is slate-grey skin discoloration related to sun exposure. Patients should be counseled on the importance of sun protection while on treatment.
- B: Corneal micro-deposits are a common adverse effect, which usually resolve on cessation of treatment. Other more significant ocular complications may rarely occur (e.g. optic neuropathy).
- C: Due to the long half-life of amiodarone, occasional missed doses are unlikely to have a significant effect on serum levels or treatment efficacy.
- D: Pulmonary toxicity is an important adverse effect of amiodarone therapy, and patients should be counseled to report respiratory symptoms early.
- E: Amiodarone has numerous interactions with other drugs; patients should be warned to check with a doctor/pharmacist before taking any new medication.

Answer 6: E

(See Ch. 13, Section 13.1)

- A: There is no association with increased stroke risk.
- B: Osteonecrosis of the jaw is a recognized but rare adverse effect of bisphosphonate treatment. It is more common with more potent agents (e.g. Zolendronate). Patients should ensure good oral and dental hygiene.
- C: Bisphosphonates should never be taken before sleep or in a supine position due to the risk of oesophageal irritation.
- D: Risedronate may be taken either daily (at low dose) or weekly for the treatment of osteoporosis.
- E: Bisphosphonates may cause oesophageal irritation or ulceration – taking them with a glass of water reduces the risk. They have very low bioavailability when taken orally, which is further reduced by the presence of food in the stomach.

21 Calculation skills

CASE PRESENTATION 1

You are working in a critical care department and are required to make up a syringe of metaraminol for infusion. The protocol requires you to dilute 1 mL of a 10 mg/mL ampoule into 50 mL of normal saline.

Calculation 1

What is the final concentration expressed in micrograms/mL?

CASE PRESENTATION 2

A patient on your ward has gone into pulseless electrical activity (PEA) cardiac arrest and the resuscitation team decides to administer 1 mg of adrenaline. You open the cardiac arrest box and find a 10-mL ampoule of adrenaline 1:10,000.

Calculation 2

What volume of adrenaline must be given?

CASE PRESENTATION 3

On a night shift, the nurses ring you to inform that an elderly patient who is NBM requires continuation of her maintenance fluids. You prescribe 1L over 12 hours but find that there are no IV trained nurses on the ward and there are no infusion pumps available, as they are all being used.

Calculation 3

A standard giving set delivers 20 drops/mL. How many drops/min do you need to set the infusion to?

CASE PRESENTATION 4

During a busy night shift in the ED, you attend to a victim of a knife attack who has multiple superficial lacerations that require suturing. Knowing that the maximum safe dose of lidocaine is 3 mg/kg (ideal body weight) you are concerned that you may require more local anaesthetic than the maximum dose. The patient weighs 70 kilograms.

Calculation 4

Given that the lidocaine available is in 1% ampoules, what is the maximum dose you may administer this patient expressed in mL?

CASE PRESENTATION 5

An elderly patient with epilepsy has become dysphagic and cannot swallow her phenytoin capsules. You decide to change her to the suspension formulation. The pharmacist has left a reminder that phenytoin suspension and capsules are not bioequivalent and that a 100-mg phenytoin capsule ≈ 92 mg phenytoin suspension.

Calculation 5

Given her capsule dose is 250 mg, how many mL of the 30 mg/5 mL suspension will you prescribe for the patient?

CASE PRESENTATION 6

You are doing a taster day with an anaesthetist who asks you to make up a remifentanil infusion pump. It's the second case of the day, similar to the first, and you know that for the previous patient the anaesthetist used a 50 mL syringe with a remifentanil concentration of 40 micrograms/mL. The anaesthetist would like 'the same as before' for this patient.

Calculation 6

How many mg of remifentanil do you need to ask the nurse for?

CASE PRESENTATION 7

During your oncology placement you are asked to prescribe the docetaxal for a patient with breast cancer. Following the local protocols you work out her body surface area (BSA) to prescribe the recommended dosage at 75 mg/m².

$$\text{BSA (m}^2\text{) (Mosteller method)} = \text{square root of (height [cm]} \times \text{weight [kg]/3600)}$$

$$\text{Weight = 70 kg; height = 159 cm}$$

Calculation 7

What is the correct dosage of docetaxal for this patient?

CASE PRESENTATION 8

Working in the ED you attend a patient who has taken a significant overdose of paracetamol. She is slim, at 50 kg, which you reason is her ideal body weight.

You decide you need to prescribe her acetylcysteine and look up the local regimen. You find you need to prescribe:

- 150 mg/kg in the first hour added to 200 mL of 5% dextrose
- 50 mg/kg in the next 4 hours added to 500 mL of 5% dextrose
- 100 mg/kg in the subsequent 16 hours added to 1 L of 5% dextrose

Acetylcysteine is available in 200 mg/mL ampoules.

Calculation 8

How many mL of acetylcysteine do you need to add to each bag?

ANSWERS

Answer 1: *200 micrograms/mL*

Workings:

$$10 \text{ mg in } 50 \text{ mL} = 1 \text{ mg in } 5 \text{ mL} = 0.2 \text{ mg/mL} = 200 \text{ micrograms/mL}$$

Answer 2: *10 mL*

Workings:

$$\text{Adrenaline } 1{:}10{,}000 = 1 \text{ g in } 10{,}000 \text{ mL (or} \equiv 1000 \text{ mg in } 10{,}000 \text{ mL)}$$
$$\text{Divide by } 1000 = 1 \text{ mg in } 10 \text{ mL}$$

Answer 3: *27.8 mL*

Workings:

$$1000/12 = 83.33 \text{ mL/hr}$$
$$83.33/60 = 1.39 \text{ mL/min}$$
$$1.39 \times 20 = 27.8 \text{ drops/minute}$$

N.B.: In reality you would aim for 30 drops/min, i.e. 1 every 2 seconds.

Answer 4: *21 mL*

Workings:

$$\text{Maximum patient dose} = 70 \text{ kg} \times 3 \text{ mg/kg} = 210 \text{ mg}$$
$$1\% = 1 \text{ g in } 100 \text{ mL (or } 1000 \text{ mg in } 100 \text{ mL} \equiv 10 \text{ mg/mL)}$$
$$\text{Maximum dose } 210/10 = 21 \text{ mL lidocaine } 1\%$$

Answer 5: *38.3 mL*

Workings:

There are a few ways to work out these calculations:

Dose required = (what you want/what you've got) × volume it's in

Desired suspension dose = 92/100 × 250 = 230 mg

Dose in mL = 230/30 × 5 ≈ 38.3 mL

Answer 6: *2 mg*

Workings:

40 micrograms/mL × 50 mL = 2000 micrograms

Amount required is 2 mg (≡ 2000 micrograms)

Answer 7: *132 mg*

Workings:

$$\sqrt{(159 \times 70/3600)}$$

~ 1.76 × 75 = 132 mg

Answer 8: *First hour 37.5 mL, next 4 hours 12.5 mL, next 16 hours 25 mL*

Workings:

First hour: 50 kg × 150 mg/kg = 7500 mg

7500 mg/200 mg/mL = 37.5 mL

Next 4 hours: 50 kg × 50 mg/kg = 2500 mg

2500 mg/200 mg/mL = 12.5 mL

Next 16 hours: 50 kg × 100 mg/kg = 5000 mg

5000 mg/200 mg/mL = 25 mL

22 Drug monitoring

CASE PRESENTATION 1

A 70-year-old man is admitted with a 7-day history of increasing shortness of breath, palpitations and abdominal pain. He is found to be in atrial fibrillation and congestive cardiac failure with oedema, hepatomegaly and a raised jugular venous pressure. He is initiated on digoxin and bumetanide.

Question 1

The most relevant measure of improvement in heart failure is:

MONITORING OPTIONS

A. A fall in blood pressure
B. A fall in body weight
C. A fall in heart rate
D. A reduction in liver size
E. Clearance of congestion on a chest x-ray

CASE PRESENTATION 2

A 24-year-old patient presents to the ED with abdominal pain and vomiting. You discover that she is a non-concordant type 1 diabetic and a diagnosis of DKA is made. Her haemodynamic parameters are within normal limits. You are aware of the local protocols and initiate 500 mL normal saline over 15 minutes and a weight-adjusted insulin sliding scale.

Question 2

What is the most reliable early indicator of hypovolaemic shock in the patient?

MONITORING OPTIONS

A. Hypotension
B. Orthostatic hypotension
C. Raised capillary refill time
D. Tachycardia
E. Tachypnoea

CASE PRESENTATION 3

A 34-year-old known asthmatic is admitted to your ED with an exacerbation of asthma. You review her an hour after admission to find her somewhat improved and keen to go home.

Question 3

Which of these parameters/scenarios would allow you to consider the potential of discharge at this point, and does not mandate an admission to hospital?

MONITORING OPTIONS

A. A normal $PaCO_2$ on admission
B. A PEF of 36% predicted on admission
C. An SpO_2 of 91% on admission
D. Cyanosis on admission
E. GCS 11 on admission (E3 V3 M5)

CASE PRESENTATION 4

An elderly woman with atrial fibrillation is on your ward for optimization of her heart failure medication. On your ward round you are told by the nursing staff that she has become tachycardic and increasingly tachypnoeic overnight. Her oxygen saturations are 96% on air, BP 100/50, HR 120 irregular. Her current medications are warfarin, digoxin, bumetanide, spironolactone and ramipril.

Question 4

After ABCDE assessment and management, what should be your initial immediate investigation to aid diagnosis and further management?

MONITORING OPTIONS

A. Chest X-ray
B. Digoxin levels
C. ECG
D. INR
E. Serum U+E

CASE PRESENTATION 5

A 65-year-old woman is admitted to your surgical ward for acute cholecystitis, and is initiated on antibiotics. She is currently taking warfarin for a DVT, and her INR from the ED is 1.9. Your consultant says he wants to operate as soon as her INR drops below 1.5 and prescribes some vitamin K.

Question 5

How many hours after the vitamin K administration should you take an initial blood sample?

MONITORING OPTIONS

A. 1 hour
B. 2 hours
C. 6 hours
D. 12 hours
E. 24 hours

CASE PRESENTATION 6

A 47-year-old woman on your urology ward is initiated on gentamicin for a resistant urinary tract infection. After 3 days of therapy the consultant is concerned the patient is experiencing gentamicin toxicity.

Question 6

Which of these abnormalities is most commonly discovered in those with gentamicin toxicity?

MONITORING OPTIONS

A. Anaemia
B. Neutropaenia
C. Raised bilirubin
D. Raised blood urea nitrogen (BUN)
E. Thrombocytopaenia

CASE PRESENTATION 7

A 31-year-old pregnant woman is initiated on therapeutic enoxaparin for treatment of a DVT. She is otherwise fit and well and no anomalies are discovered during diagnostic investigations.

Question 7

Which of the following options would you routinely monitor to assess for an immune mediated complication of her treatment?

MONITORING OPTIONS

A. Haemoglobin
B. Lymphocytes
C. Mean corpuscular volume
D. Neutrophils
E. Platelets

Self-assessment

CASE PRESENTATION 8

A 65-year-old male presents to the ED with a temporal headache. He has previously been diagnosed with temporal arteritis and is currently on a reducing dose of prednisolone. He is under the rheumatology team at your hospital, and all previous blood test results are available to you.

Question 8

Which of the following parameters is the most appropriate for assessing whether this is an acute progression of his disease process?

MONITORING OPTIONS

A. C-reactive protein (CRP)
B. Erythrocyte sedimentation rate
C. Ferritin
D. Fibrinogen
E. White cell count

ANSWERS

Answer 1: B

- A: Not a reliable indicator of cardiac function or fluid status.
- B: Short-term weight changes reliably reflect fluid shifts in heart failure.
- C: This may indicate control of the AF and subsequent improvement in cardiac output but is not a measure of improvement in heart failure.
- D: Not a reliable indicator of heart function or fluid status.
- E: Not a reliable indicator of heart function or fluid status.

Answer 2: B

(See Ch. 15, MICRO-facts: fluid status assessment)
- A: In young adults this is a late sign of hypovolaemia.
- B: An early indicator of hypovolaemia, often associated with dizziness on standing.
- C: May be an early indicator of shock, but is unreliable as a clinical sign.
- D: Young adults may only present with significant tachycardia in moderate hypovolaemic shock.
- E: A later change in hypovolaemic shock. Unreliable here as may be raised due to acidosis.

Answer 3: B

(See BTS guidance for asthma; also see Ch. 6)
- A: This is associated with life-threatening asthma and warrants admission.
- B: PEF 33.50% is associated with an acute severe exacerbation. If her PEF is >75% best or predicted greater than an hour after admission and she is clinically improved, you may consider discharge.

- C: Saturations <92% on admission is associated with life-threatening asthma and warrants admission.
- D: This is associated with life-threatening asthma and warrants admission.
- E: Exhaustion or altered conscious level is associated with life-threatening asthma and warrants admission.

Answer 4: C

- A: Decompensation of heart failure is likely and pulmonary oedema may be present. This will take time to organize and is unlikely to change your initial management based on clinical findings.
- B: Will take time to return and therefore not alter initial management. ECG may guide diagnosis of potential digoxin toxicity.
- C: Risk of hyperkalaemia with ACE inhibitors and spironolactone despite bumetanide use. Possible digoxin toxicity. An ECG can be done quickly on the ward. Diagnostic changes may be found in both above conditions, allowing treatment to be instigated rapidly.
- D: Unlikely to be helpful.
- E: Will take time to return and therefore not alter initial management. ECG may show changes associated with electrolyte disturbances. Note an arterial gas may be helpful and achieved rapidly, and often gives a potassium level.

Answer 5: C

- A: Not enough time allowed to pass.
- B: Not enough time allowed to pass.
- C: Vitamin K may have some effect within around 6 hours post administration, though a significant drop may not be seen for around 24 hours. As this woman needs urgent surgery and has a marginally high INR, around 6 hours for the initial blood test is reasonable.
- D: Too long for initial sample in this case.
- E: Too long for initial sample in this case.

Answer 6: D

- A: Rarely associated with blood dyscrasias.
- B: Rarely associated with blood dyscrasias.
- C: No frequent association with liver dysfunction.
- D: Gentamicin accumulation is strongly associated with nephrotoxicity, in particular acute tubular necrosis (ATN). A raised BUN and serum creatinine are found in ATN.
- E: Rarely associated with blood dyscrasias.

Answer 7: E

- A: Anaemia may be caused by bleeding, but is not immune mediated.
- B: Not commonly affected by heparin use.

- C: Not commonly affected by heparin use.
- D: Not commonly affected by heparin use.
- E: Heparin and low molecular weight heparins are associated with HIT (heparin-induced thrombocytopaenia) (see Ch. 14, Section 14.1).

Answer 8: A

- A: An acute-phase protein used to monitor progression in acute temporal arteritis. Levels will increase more rapidly compared to ESR. Common use as an acute inflammatory marker means previous levels will often be available for comparison.
- B: Useful in initial diagnosis and for follow-up monitoring of the disease process. It is however less useful for monitoring and diagnosis in the acute phase of known disease.
- C: Forms part of an iron profile, however also an acute-phase protein. Not routinely used for monitoring.
- D: Not used for the monitoring of rheumatological conditions.
- E: May take days to increase.

Data interpretation

CASE PRESENTATION 1

On your morning ward round with the consultant you review an elderly patient who is taking her tablets and finishing her breakfast. She is alert and well and awaiting social care for discharge. You notice she has a persistent tachycardia of 90–110 bpm, and are aware she is taking 125 micrograms of digoxin daily for atrial fibrillation. Your consultant suggests you do a digoxin level, which you do an hour later after you have finished the morning round. By late afternoon the level comes back as 2.2 micrograms/L (normal range 0.8–2).

Question 1

What is the correct course of action?

DECISION OPTIONS

A. Decrease the dose to 62.5 micrograms.
B. Increase the dose to 187.5 micrograms for clinical effect.
C. Make no alteration to the dose.
D. Repeat the blood test now.
E. Repeat the blood test the following day after rounds to re-check the level.

CASE PRESENTATION 2

You are on call one afternoon and are asked to check and act upon blood results for a 32-year-old woman admitted to an orthopaedic ward. She has severe asthma and is a smoker who was started on theophylline M/R 175 mg BD 2 weeks previously and has been taking them as prescribed. Early that morning before drug rounds she had become acutely short of breath, and trough theophylline levels were sent as recommended by the respiratory registrar at his review. You review the patient who is now much improved. When you check the levels you find they are 6 mg/L (range 10–20).

Question 2

What is the correct course of action?

DECISION OPTIONS

A. Increase the theophylline M/R to 350 mg BD.
B. Increase the theophylline M/R to 250 mg BD.
C. Increase the theophylline M/R to 200 mg BD.
D. Increase the theophylline M/R to 175 mg TDS.
E. Decrease the dose to theophylline M/R 200 mg OD.

CASE PRESENTATION 3

A 76-year-old male with COPD is admitted under the respiratory team with an infective exacerbation of COPD. You assess him at the post-take ward round the following morning and note the treatments he has received. He was administered 30 mg of prednisolone and 200 mg of doxycycline in the ED, and has taken 30 mg prednisolone and 100 mg of doxycycline this morning. The patient says he feels about the same, maybe a touch better. Below is a comparison of his ED blood results and the results from this morning's sample:

BLOOD TEST	ED RESULT	MORNING SAMPLE
WCC ($4.0–11 \times 10^9$/l)	15.9	20.1
Neutrophils ($2.0–7.5 \times 10^9$/L)	14.3	18.9
Lymphocytes ($1.3–3.5 \times 10^9$/L)	1.3	0.9
CRP (<5 mg/L)	12.4	9.3

Question 3

From the blood results, what is the appropriate course of action?

DECISION OPTIONS

A. Change to co-amoxiclav 1.2 g TDS, IV.
B. Change to co-amoxiclav 625 mg TDS, Oral.
C. Change to Tazocin 4.5 g TDS, IV.
D. Increase the doxycycline dose to 100 mg BD.
E. Make no change to above treatments.

CASE PRESENTATION 4

A 56-year-old male is admitted under medicine by his GP. He has a history of recurrent DVT and is on lifelong warfarin. He attended his GP today after cutting himself shaving and noting that he was unable to stop the bleeding. His INR result is 7.9.

Question 4

What is the correct course of action?

DECISION OPTIONS

A. Stop warfarin and administer dried prothrombin complex (e.g. Beriplex®).
B. Stop warfarin and administer fresh frozen plasma 15 mL/kg.
C. Stop warfarin and administer vitamin K 10 mg, IV.
D. Stop warfarin and administer vitamin K 1 mg, IV.
E. Stop warfarin and repeat INR the following day.

CASE PRESENTATION 5

A normally fit and well 23-year-old woman is admitted to your urology ward with acute kidney injury. She had presented to her GP 2 days earlier with dysuria and he had initiated nitrofurantoin 50 mg QDS for a urinary tract infection (UTI). The U+Es she had taken on that day showed a creatinine of 63. Since then she had been vomiting and hadn't been drinking much though she was still able to take her tablets. She has no signs of an ascending UTI. U+Es taken today show a creatinine of 130.

Question 5

What is the correct course of action?

DECISION OPTIONS

A. Start IV fluids and continue on current dose of nitrofurantoin.
B. Start IV fluids and decrease dose of nitrofurantoin to 50 mg TDS.
C. Start IV fluids and decrease dose of nitrofurantoin to 50 mg BD.
D. Start IV fluids and decrease dose of nitrofurantoin to 50 mg daily.
E. Start IV fluids and select alternative antibiotic.

CASE PRESENTATION 6

On your GP rotation a woman presents with a 1-week history of mild muscle weakness. There are no other concerning features and she is otherwise asymptomatic. You order a variety of investigations and inform her you'll call her the following day with the results. Her blood results return indicating a serum potassium of 5.5 mmol/L (previous 4.1 mmol/L). Her ECG is unremarkable. She has a history of mild LVF and angina, and was recently started on ramipril. Other medications include furosemide, isosorbide mononitrate, amiloride and aspirin.

Question 6

What is the correct course of action?

DECISION OPTIONS

A. Increase furosemide.
B. No change needed.

C. Stop amiloride.
D. Stop isosorbide mononitrate.
E. Stop ramipril.

ANSWERS

Answer 1: D

- A: This would be inappropriate due to timing of blood test (see below).
- B: This would be unwise upon receipt of a high level, although this is likely the correct course of action following a correctly timed blood test (see below).
- C: This would be inappropriate due to timing of blood test (see below).
- D: Digoxin levels should be taken at least 6–8 hours post dose. Late afternoon is likely to be an acceptable time for the level to be representative of serum concentration and allow appropriate dose alteration.
- E: This would likely give the same result.

Answer 2: A

- A: The levels are sub-therapeutic and the patient will be at steady state having received 2 weeks of therapy. Due to predictable first-order metabolism doubling the dose should give a level within therapeutic range. As a smoker she is likely to require higher doses due to increased metabolism (see Ch. 6).
- B: Unlikely to represent sufficient increase.
- C: Unlikely to represent sufficient increase.
- D: These modified release preparations are designed for 12-hourly administration.
- E: Inappropriate dose reduction.

Answer 3: E

- A: No indication to change therapy.
- B: No indication to change therapy.
- C: No indication to change therapy.
- D: No indication to increase dose.
- E: Patient has not deteriorated and may have improved. CRP is an acute-phase protein and the reduction is most likely to represent an improvement in the patient's condition. Corticosteroids may be associated with a neutrophilia and lymphopenia which may well account for these changes in the FBC.

Answer 4: D

- A: Indicated with major bleeding where rapid reversal is required. May be indicated even if INR within normal range.

- B: Indicated with major bleeding where rapid reversal is required. May be indicated even if INR within normal range. Less effective than dried prothrombin complex.
- C: High dose. Often used in pathological coagulopathy (such as hepatic disease). Not normally indicated in warfarin reversal as this renders warfarin ineffective for several days. If concern is major bleeding, then other options discussed above are normally more suitable.
- D: With INR <8 and minor bleeding, low-dose vitamin K (1–5 mg) is indicated. Local policies may vary as to preference for IV/oral, as both are effective. 1–2 mg is commonly used as this will start to reduce INR within 6–8 hours (maximum effect 24–48 hours) and will allow warfarin to be re-prescribed within days of treatment.
- E: Not appropriate with active bleeding.

Answer 5: E

- A: Nitrofurantoin requires an eGFR >60 mL/min/1.73 m² in order to provide adequate urinary concentrations to treat UTIs (this equates to a creatinine of approximately 100 in a white female). Renal failure also increases risk of peripheral neuropathy with nitrofurantoin.
- B: See answer A.
- C: See answer A.
- D: See answer A.
- E: IV fluids are indicated due to inadequate fluid intake. Nitrofurantoin must be changed to an alternative as explained above.

Answer 6: C

- A: May reduce potassium levels, but no indication to increase loop diuretic dose.
- B: Patient complains of symptomatic hyperkalaemia and change is warranted.
- C: Amiloride is a weak diuretic, normally co-administered with furosemide to prevent hypokalaemia. Minimal symptomatic improvement, therefore this should be stopped.
- D: Isosorbide mononitrate has no impact on potassium levels.
- E: Ramipril in combination with amiloride is the likely culprit. However it provides symptomatic relief in LVF and is indicated in this patient. It should be continued.

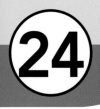

Planning management

CASE PRESENTATION 1

A 75-year-old woman is admitted with worsening breathlessness and cough. She was recently admitted with similar symptoms.

- PMH: Myocardial infarction, hypertension.
- DH: Furosemide 40 mg daily, ramipril 5 mg daily, aspirin 75 mg daily.
- On examination: Temperature 36.7, HR 110/min regular, BP 110/52 mmHg, RR 32/min, oxygen sat 85% on room air. Chest examination reveals bilateral basal crackles and cardiac auscultation reveals a gallop rhythm.
- Investigations: CXR shows grossly congested lung fields and cardiomegaly.

Question 1

Select the *most appropriate* management option at this stage.

MANAGEMENT OPTIONS

A. 0.9% saline 500 mL IV
B. Bisoprolol 5 mg orally
C. Co-amoxiclav 1.2 g IV
D. Furosemide 50 mg IV
E. Salbutamol 5 mg via nebulizer

CASE PRESENTATION 2

A 62-year-old man presents to the ED with reduced consciousness.

- PMH: Advanced prostate cancer.
- DH: Slow-release morphine 20 mg twice-daily, liquid morphine 10 mg as required, ibuprofen 400 mg 8-hourly, omeprazole 20 mg daily.
- On examination: HR 56/min and regular, RR 8/min, oxygen sat 95% on room air, BP 129/67. GCS 9/15 (E2V3M4), blood glucose 6.1 mmol/L. Pupils pinpoint and unreactive.

Question 2

Select the *most appropriate* management option at this stage.

MANAGEMENT OPTIONS

A. 50% glucose 50 mL IV
B. Flumezenil 200 micrograms
C. Naloxone 200 micrograms
D. Oxygen 15 L/min via non-rebreathe mask
E. Paracetamol 1 g IV

CASE PRESENTATION 3

A 19-year-old man with known asthma is seen in the outpatient clinic. He is currently using an inhaled beta-agonist to treat his symptoms as required. He is using his inhaler around twice a week.

- DH: Salbutamol 400 micrograms inhaled PRN.
- SH: Smokes ~5 cigarettes/day.
- On examination: RR 18/min, HR 65/min, BP125/60. Oxygen sat 99% on room air. Chest examination: very mild expiratory wheeze.

Question 3

Select the *most appropriate* management option at this stage.

MANAGEMENT OPTIONS

A. Beclometasone 200 micrograms inhaled 12-hourly
B. Montelukast 10 mg orally daily
C. Prednisolone 40 mg daily for 5 days
D. Salmeterol 100 μg inhaled 12-hourly
E. Theophylline SR 250 mg 12-hourly

CASE PRESENTATION 4

A 36-year-old woman is admitted with acute onset shortness of breath and chest pains. She has recently taken a long haul flight back from Thailand.

- PMH: Appendectomy age 21 yrs.
- DH: Combined oral contraceptive pill.
- SH: Light drinker.
- On examination: Weight 60 kg. RR 32/min, HR 98/min, BP130/75. Oxygen sat 98% on 4 L/min oxygen. Chest examination: clear. Swollen left calf.
- Investigations: CXR clear. CTPA: left upper lobe sub-segmental pulmonary embolus. Serum creatinine 70 μmol/L, Hb 13.1 g/L, platelets 260×10^9.

Question 4

Select the *most appropriate* management option at this stage.

MANAGEMENT OPTIONS

A. Danaparoid 750 IU subcutaneously 12-hourly
B. Enoxaparin 1.5 mg/kg subcutaneously daily
C. Enoxaparin 40 mg subcutaneously daily
D. Unfractionated heparin 5000 IU subcutaneously 12-hourly
E. Warfarin loading

ANSWERS

Answer 1: D

- A: There is evidence of fluid overload and further IV fluid is likely to be detrimental.
- B: Beta-blockers are of use in the long-term management of heart failure but are contraindicated in acute left ventricular failure as they reduce heart rate and contractility, further impairing cardiac output.
- C: No evidence of infection.
- D: This patient has good evidence of left ventricular failure with pulmonary oedema. An IV diuretic is indicated (see Ch. 5, Section 5.4).
- E: Pulmonary oedema due to LVF can result in a degree of small airway obstruction, but this is not the primary problem and bronchodilators will not significantly help the patient.

Answer 2: C

- A: This patient has normal blood glucose and does not require intravenous glucose.
- B: Flumazenil is used in benzodiazepine overdose.
- C: This patient has a history and features suggesting opioid toxicity. Naloxone should be administered urgently to reverse the effects of opioid overdose, and the patient's conscious level should improve rapidly (see Ch. 10, Section 10.4).
- D: The patient has a depressed respiratory rate and reduced consciousness, although oxygen saturations are currently acceptable. Oxygen may be required as part of the management of a patient with reduced consciousness.
- E: Pain is not the primary concern here.

Answer 3: A

- A: The next step up from simple reliever therapy in the stepwise management of asthma is to add a regular inhaled corticosteroid (ICS) such as beclometasone. The dose of this can be increased as required to achieve good control of symptoms (see Ch. 6, Section 6.1).
- B: Not indicated at this stage.
- C: Indicated in an acute exacerbation of asthma.

- D: An inhaled long-acting beta agonist may be required to control this man's asthma, but this is currently skipping a step in the stepwise treatment of asthma.
- E: Not indicated at this stage.

Answer 4: B

- A: Danaparoid is used in the prophylaxis and treatment of VTE in patients with HIT.
- B: This patient has a VTE and requires therapeutic anticoagulation. The most appropriate agent initially is a LMWH such as enoxaparin. This is given at a therapeutic dose of 1.5 mg/kg once daily until alternative oral anticoagulation (usually warfarin) reaches a therapeutic level (see Ch. 14, Section 14.1).
- C: This is the prophylactic dose.
- D: Unfractionated heparin is now usually reserved for prophylaxis and treatment of VTE in patients in whom LMWHs are contraindicated.
- E: Oral vitamin K antagonists such as warfarin initially have a pro-thrombotic effect, and so they should not be initiated without alternative anticoagulation in most cases.

25

Prescription review

CASE PRESENTATION 1

A 64-year-old woman with ischaemic heart disease and heart failure has been admitted for an elective cataract surgery. Her routine blood tests on admission reveal moderate renal impairment with a serum creatinine of 306 μmol/L. Her current regular medications are listed below.

CURRENT PRESCRIPTIONS

A. Aspirin 75 mg orally daily
B. Bisoprolol 5 mg orally daily
C. Digoxin 125 mg orally daily
D. Furosemide 40 mg orally twice daily (asymmetric dosing)
E. Ibuprofen 400 mg orally 8-hourly
F. Omeprazole 20 mg orally daily
G. Paracetamol 1 g orally 6-hourly
H. Ramipril 5 mg orally daily

Question 1A
Select the ONE drug that is prescribed incorrectly.

Question 1B
Select the THREE drugs that are *most likely* to be contributing to her renal impairment.

CASE PRESENTATION 2

A 71-year-old woman is admitted with a history of cough and increasing breathlessness. She has been treated for a chest infection with oral antibiotics by her GP. She has also recently been started on an agent to reduce her serum cholesterol, and a new drug to control her heart rate.
- PMH: Atrial fibrillation, osteoarthritis, previous MI.
- Examination: HR 49 and irregular, BP 90/45, crepitations at right lung base.
- Investigations: WCC 16.4×10^9, U+Es normal range, INR 6.1.
- Her currently prescribed medications are listed below.

CURRENT PRESCRIPTIONS

A. Atenolol 50 mg orally daily
B. Atorvastatin 40 mg orally at night
C. Co-codamol 8/500 2 tabs orally 4-hourly as required
D. Diltiazem 90 mg orally 12-hourly
E. Erythromycin 500 mg orally 12-hourly for 5 days
F. Quinine sulphate 300 mg orally at night
G. Warfarin 3 mg orally daily

Question 2A

Select the TWO drugs that are *most likely* to have contributed to the patients raised INR.

Question 2B

Select the TWO drugs that should not normally be prescribed together.

CASE PRESENTATION 3

A 46-year-old man with polycystic kidney disease is admitted with a non-ST elevation MI (NSTEMI). During his admission he develops hospital-acquired pneumonia requiring IV antibiotics. He is not currently on renal replacement therapy.

- Investigations: Serum creatinine 550 µmol/L, creatinine clearance 14 mL/min.
- His currently prescribed medications are listed below.

CURRENT PRESCRIPTIONS

A. Aspirin 300 mg orally daily
B. Atorvastatin 80 mg orally daily
C. Bisoprolol 2.5 mg orally 12-hourly
D. Calcium carbonate 500 mg orally 8-hourly
E. Clopidogrel 300 mg orally daily
F. Dalteparin 5000 units subcutaneously daily
G. Piperacillin-tazobactam 4.5 g IV 8-hourly for 5 days
H. Ramipril 10 mg orally daily

Question 3A

Select the TWO drugs that must be prescribed at a reduced dose in severe renal impairment.

Question 3B

Select the ONE drug that has been prescribed incorrectly.

CASE PRESENTATION 4

A 78-year-old man is seen by his GP for a medication review. He mentions that he has recently been having difficulty passing urine. He was started on a new inhaler six weeks ago. He also admits to a dry mouth.

- PMH: Ischaemic heart disease, heart failure, severe COPD.
- Examination: HR 87/min and regular, BP 124/78, oxygen sat 89% on room air, chest: globally reduced air entry, sparse crepitations. Oral thrush noted.
- Investigations: Na^+136, K^+6.3, urea 6.7, creatinine 105.
- His current regular medications are listed below.

CURRENT PRESCRIPTIONS

A. Aspirin 75 mg orally daily
B. Atorvastatin 40 mg orally daily
C. Carvedilol 6.25 mg orally 12-hourly
D. Furosemide 40 mg orally daily
E. Ramipril 5 mg orally daily
F. Salbutamol 400 micrograms inhaled as needed
G. Salmeterol 50 micrograms/fluticasone 250 micrograms 2 puffs inhaled 12-hourly
H. Spironolactone 12.5 mg orally daily
 I. Theophylline sustained release 250 mg orally 12-hourly
J. Tiotropium 18 micrograms inhaled daily

Question 4A

Select the ONE drug that is the *most likely* to have caused his dry mouth and difficulty with micturition.

Question 4B

Select the TWO drugs that are *most likely* to be contributing to his hyperkalaemia.

Question 4C

Select the ONE drug that is *most likely* to have resulted in his oral candidiasis.

CASE PRESENTATION 5

A 67-year-old woman is recovering in hospital 1 week after an elective knee replacement. She has developed dysuria and confusion and is diagnosed with a urinary tract infection.

- PMH: Type 2 diabetes mellitus, angina, heart failure.
- Her currently prescribed medications are listed below.

CURRENT PRESCRIPTIONS

A. Amlodipine 10 mg orally daily
B. Bisoprolol 2.5 mg orally daily
C. Furosemide 40 mg orally 12-hourly
D. Isosorbide mononitrate 20 mg orally 12-hourly
E. Lisinopril 10 mg orally daily
F. Mixtard 15 U subcutaneously 12-hourly
G. Paracetamol 1 g orally 4-hourly as required
H. Trimethoprim 200 mg orally 12-hourly

Question 5A

Select the FIVE drugs that have been prescribed incorrectly or sub-optimally.

CASE PRESENTATION 6

A 37-year-old man with known epilepsy is admitted with a 5-day history of confusion. He has recently been started on new pain medication for lower back pain, and is receiving a course of treatment for a fungal skin infection.

- PMH: Idiopathic generalized epilepsy, chronic low back pain.
- Examination: Nystagmus, mild limb ataxia. Haemodynamically stable.
- Investigations: U+E normal ranges, serum phenytoin level 42 µg/L (normal range 10–20 µg/L).
- His currently prescribed medications are listed below.

CURRENT PRESCRIPTIONS

A. Co-codamol 8/500 2 tabs orally 6-hourly
B. Fluconazole 50 mg orally daily for 14 days
C. Folic acid 5 mg orally daily
D. Ibuprofen 400 mg orally 8-hourly
E. Omeprazole 20 mg orally daily
F. Paracetamol 1 g orally 6-hourly
G. Phenytoin 300 mg orally daily

Question 6A

Select the TWO drugs that are *most likely* to have contributed to the raised serum phenytoin level.

Question 6B

Select TWO other drugs that have been prescribed incorrectly or in error.

CASE PRESENTATION 7

A 71-year-old woman is reviewed by her GP after complaining of lethargy and a sore throat. She was treated a few days earlier for a urinary tract infection.

- PMH: Rheumatoid arthritis, hypertension.
- Examination: HR 105/min and regular, BP 92/48, oxygen sat 98% on room air, temperature 37.5°C.
- Investigations: Hb 8.2 g/L, WCC 2.1 × 10⁹, neutrophils 0.9 × 10⁹, platelets 89 × 10⁹, U+Es normal range.
- Her current regular medications are listed below.

CURRENT MEDICATIONS

A. Alendronate 30 mg orally once-weekly
B. Bendroflumethiazide 2.5 mg orally daily
C. Calcium carbonate 500 mg orally daily
D. Diclofenac 50 mg TDS orally 8-hourly
E. Lisinopril 5 mg daily
F. Sulfasalazine 1 g orally daily
G. Trimethoprim 200 mg orally 12-hourly for 3 days

Question 7A

Select the TWO drugs *most likely* to have contributed to her full blood count result.

Question 7B

Select the TWO drugs *most likely* to have contributed to her hypotension.

CASE PRESENTATION 8

A 56-year-old man weighing 70 kg is admitted with a 1-day history of confusion and fevers. He has suffered a single generalized tonic clonic seizure.

- PMH: Hypercholesterolaemia, analphyactic reaction to penicillin.
- Investigations: CSF glucose 2.1 mmol/L (serum 4.4 mmol/L), protein 0.52 g/L, neutrophils 24, lymphocytes 67, Gram stain negative. Blood tests: ALT 280, AST 233, ALP 157, GGT 131, bilirubin 35, albumin 25.
- His currently prescribed medications are listed below.

CURRENT MEDICATIONS

A. Aciclovir 70 mg IV 8-hourly for 10 days
B. Aspirin 75 mg orally daily
C. Cefotaxime 2 g IV 6-hourly for 7 days
D. Haloperidol 2.5 mg orally at night
E. Omeprazole 20 mg orally daily
F. Simvastatin 40 mg orally at night
G. Sodium valproate sustained-release 300 mg orally 12-hourly

Question 8A

Select the TWO drugs that are prescribed incorrectly or at the wrong dose.

Question 8B

Select the TWO drugs that are *most likely* to be contributing to his elevated liver enzymes.

ANSWERS

Answer 1A: C

- Digoxin is a cardiac glycoside which slows the heart rate and increases cardiac contractility. It is normally prescribed as a maintenance dose of 62.5 to 250 micrograms daily. 125 mg is a huge overdose. In addition, given the patient's renal impairment, it is likely that there has been accumulation of digoxin leading to supra-therapeutic serum levels. The patient's digoxin level should be checked before administering further doses.

Answer 1B: D, E, H

(See Ch. 10, Section 10.3)

- Furosemide is loop diuretic and may reduce renal perfusion due to volume depletion.
- Ibuprofen is an NSAID, and reduction in prostaglandin production due to non-selective COX antagonism results in constriction of the afferent glomerular arteriole and reduced perfusion.
- Ramipril is an ACE-inhibitor, and the reduction in angiotensin II production results in reduced glomerular perfusion.
- All of these mechanisms are likely to result in renal impairment with an increase in serum creatinine.

Answer 2A: B, E

- Atorvastatin is a statin and inhibits the cytochrome P450 group of liver enzymes that metabolize warfarin, again resulting in increased levels of active drug.
- Erythromycin is a macrolide antibiotic and binds readily to serum albumin. This may have the effect of displacing albumin-bound warfarin, thus increasing the amount of active drug in circulation and increasing the INR.

Answer 2B: A, D

(See Ch. 5, Section 5.6)

- Non-dihydropyridine calcium channel blockers (such as diltiazem) and beta receptor antagonists (such as atenolol) both act to reduce the heart rate and cardiac contractility.
- When prescribed together there may be an excessive reduction in heart rate or contractility, resulting in a dangerous drop in cardiac output.

Answer 3A: F, G

- Both penicillins (e.g. piperacillin-tazobactam) and low-molecular weight heparins (e.g. dalteparin) are primarily eliminated in the urine.
- This man has severe renal impairment with a marked reduction in creatinine clearance. Drugs with mainly renal elimination are likely to accumulate in the serum, potentially leading to significant adverse affects, and thus need to be prescribed at lower doses.

Answer 3B: C

- Bisoprolol is administered once daily, not 12-hourly.

Answer 4A: J

- Tiotropium is a long-acting anticholinergic that may cause systemic anti-muscarinic adverse effects (see Ch. 6, Section 6.1).

Answer 4B: E, H

- Ramipril is an ACE-inhibitor and so inhibits the production of angiotensin II, which normally acts to promote K^+ excretion from the renal tubules. Reduced levels of angiotensin II can result in hyperkalaemia.
- Spironolactone antagonizes the effects of aldosterone in the distal convoluted tubule, and so results in increased retention of K^+.

Answer 4C: G

- Fluticasone is a corticosteroid. Deposition via inhalation in the oropharynx and buccal cavity reduces immunity to fungal infection, particularly with *Candida* species. It is important to advise patients on correct inhaler technique and to rinse the mouth with water after administering an ICS.

Answer 5A: C, D, F, G, H

- C: Furosemide should usually be prescribed 'asymmetrically', i.e. not given late at night, to avoid the patient having to get up during the night to urinate.
- D: Patients quickly develop tolerance to the effects of nitrates, and so they should be prescribed asymmetrically to provide a 'wash-out' period so that efficacy is maintained.
- F: Mixed insulins should be prescribed by brand name and with any numbers indicating the proportions of insulins contained (e.g. Mixtard 30). The word 'units' should also be written in full rather than 'U' or 'IU'.
- G: Paracetamol may be administered 4-hourly up to a maximum of 4 g daily.
- H: Antibiotics such as trimethoprim should always be prescribed with a set course length included.

Answer 6A: B, E

- Phenytoin is metabolized by the hepatic cytochrome P450 enzyme system, which both omeprazole and fluconazole inhibit to a degree.
- Administration of these drugs to a patient receiving phenytoin may therefore lead to increased serum levels and clinical toxicity, due to reduced hepatic metabolism. A reduction in the phenytoin dose may be needed.

Answer 6B: A, F

- This patient is prescribed co-codamol and paracetamol at the same time – co-codamol contains paracetamol and so co-administration will lead to paracetamol overdose.

Answer 7A: F, G

(See Ch. 11, Section 11.1 and Ch. 7, Section 7.2)
- This patient has marrow suppression and neutropaenia.
- Sulfasalazine and trimethoprim both have anti-folate activity and may cause marrow suppression.
- Concomitant use with sulfasalazine may precipitate acute marrow suppression.

Answer 7B: B, E

- Bendroflumethiazide is thiazide diuretic and may produce hypotension due to hypovolaemia.
- Lisinopril reduces production of the potent vasoconstrictor angiotensin-II and thus results in hypotension.

Answer 8A: A, C

- For empirical treatment of viral encephalitis and bacterial meningitis the dose of aciclovir is 10 mg/kg 3 times daily, not 1 mg/kg.
- The patient has a documented anaphylactic reaction to penicillin. As such he should not receive any beta-lactam antibiotics or their derivatives (for example cephalosporins) due to the risk of cross-reactivity.

Answer 8B: F, G

- Statins such as simvastatin commonly cause insignificant rises in hepatic enzyme. They occasionally cause hepatocellular damage, usually within weeks of starting treatment.
- Sodium valproate is an anticonvulsant which may also cause elevations in hepatic enzymes as well as clinically significant hepatic damage, sometimes in an idiosyncratic manner.

26

Prescribing

QUESTIONS

BACKGROUND

- This section of self-assessment questions and answers is different to the others in this book in that it requires you to review a clinical scenario and make an appropriate prescription, thus mirroring the Prescribing Skills Assessment (PSA).
- It is designed to test:
  - Reasoning and judgement associated with the clinical scenario:
    - May be acute or chronic conditions.
    - Will require consideration of different drugs, different formulations, different routes, different doses, and different dose intervals.
  - Effective, safe and legal prescribing.
- Prescriptions must meet appropriate standards:
  - Legible, unambiguous and complete (approved name written in upper case, appropriate form and route, correct dose appropriately written without abbreviations, necessary details and instructions and signed).
- A variety of example prescription charts will be used.

QUESTION INFORMATION

- The brief scenarios below show some of the variety of prescriptions you may be asked to write.
- Instead of you writing your own prescription, examples are provided but they contain some errors.
- Initially evaluate each prescription chart and then review the corrected example chart along with the explanation for each change.

Scenario 1

Please review this prescription for an NSAID for acute back pain in a 56-year-old male smoker with hypertension. Gastrointestinal protection was also required. Has anything been omitted?

REGULAR MEDICATION															

Approved Name of Medicine		Dose		Freq	Time										
IBUPROFEN		400mg		TDS											
Additional instructions		Start date	Route		8										
		2/2/15	ORAL												
Signature	Pharmacist check	POD	Supply												
Date					14										
Print name	Bleep no.														
A. Doctor #123					22										

Approved Name of Medicine		Dose		Freq	Time										
OMEPRAZOLE		20mg		OD											
Additional instructions		Start date	Route		8										
		2/2/15	ORAL												
Signature	Pharmacist check	POD	Supply												
Date															
Print name	Bleep no.														
A. Doctor #123															

Approved Name of Medicine		Dose		Freq	Time										
Additional instructions		Start date	Route												
Signature	Pharmacist check	POD	Supply												
Print name	Bleep no.														

Scenario 2

Please review this prescription for doxycycline which is required for infective exacerbation of COPD.

REGULAR MEDICATION					

Approved Name of Medicine	Dose		Freq	Time	
DOXYCYCLINE	100mg		OD		
Additional instructions	Start date	Route	8		
	2/2/15	ORAL			
Signature	Pharmacist check	POD	Supply		
A. Doctor # 123					
Print name	Bleep no.				

Approved Name of Medicine	Dose		Freq	Time	
Additional instructions	Start date	Route			
Signature	Pharmacist check	POD	Supply		
Print name	Bleep no.				

Approved Name of Medicine	Dose		Freq	Time	
Additional instructions	Start date	Route			
Signature	Pharmacist check	POD	Supply		
Print name	Bleep no.				

Scenario 3

Please review this prescription for a PRN opioid for patient already taking regular oral paracetamol and full dose dihydrocodeine.

AS REQUIRED MEDICATION												
Approved Name of Medicine ORAMORPH	Dose 10 mg	Route ORAL	Date									
Additional instructions	Min. interval 2 hourly	Max. in 24 hours 60mg	Time									
			Dose									
Signature	Start date 2/2/15	Pharmacist check										
Print name A. Doctor # 123			Route									
Bleep no.	POD	Supply	Given									
Approved Name of Medicine	Dose	Route	Date									
Additional instructions	Min. interval	Max. in 24 hours	Time									
			Dose									
Signature	Start date	Pharmacist check										
Print name			Route									
Bleep no.	POD	Supply	Given									

Scenario 4

Please review this prescription for a loading dose of warfarin for a 40-year-old, 80-kg patient with a first episode of DVT. The patient is otherwise well.

STH WARFARIN PRESCRIPTION AND MONITORING CHART

Indication for treatment _DVT_

Target INR range _2·5 (RANGE 2-3)_ (see over)

Recommended duration of treatment (please tick):

6 weeks ☐   12 weeks ☑   6 months ☐   long term ☐

Newly starting treatment? (please tick):

Yes ☑   No ☐   (usual dose _____ mg)

INR monitored by: GP ☐   STH clinic ☐   other ☐ _____

Name: FRANCIS BACON

DOB: 2/3/45

Hosp No.: AB 1234

NHS No.:

Ward   Consultant

A1   AAB

Chronic Atrial Fibrillation (without an established thromboembolic event)
Cross through the dosing chart overleaf and follow STH Warfarin Slow Start Regimen.

Elderly Patients
1. High risk of drug interaction with warfarin due to likelihood of higher co-morbidity and polypharmacy.
2. Decision to initiate should take into account likely compliance, attendance for INR checks and risk of falling.
3. Normal ageing and/or acute ill health may require treatment to be reviewed in light of point 2 above.

Cancer Patients
Patients with active malignancy, particularly if receiving chemo/radiotherapy, should be considered for ongoing treatment with low molecular weight heparin. Discuss with oncology consultant or ask for haematology advice.

Tromboembolic Disease in Pregnancy and the Puerperium
Avoid warfarin therapy during pregnancy. Seek advice from an obstetrician on heparin treatment in pregnancy and warfarin initiation in the puerperium.

MONITORING AND DOSING GUIDANCE OVERLEAF

WARFARIN if baseline INR is greater than 1.4 seek advice from the responsible consultant.
the prescribing doctor must know the baseline INR before signing the first dose of warfarin.

Date	INR	Oral dose in milligrams (to be given at 6p)m	Signature of prescriber	Signature of administering nurse
2/2/15	Baseline	10 mg	A. Doctor #123	

Self-assessment

Scenario 5

Please review this prescription for 24 hours of maintenance fluid therapy for a 70-kg patient fasting for a procedure. He is well, euvolaemic, and has a normal electrolyte status.

RECORD OF INFUSION THERAPY

Date	Infusion fluid	Route	Volume of infusion	Additives Approved name	Additives Dose	Additives Batch No.	Rate of infusion	Start time	Prescriber's signature & bleep No.	Pharmacy	Infusion started Time	Infusion started Vol.	Infusion started By	Infusion started Check	Batch No.	Pump No.	Reason not to administ.
2/2/15	DEXTROSE	IV	1000ml	POTASSIUM CHLORIDE	20mmol		8 hours		*A. Doctor # 123*								
2/2/15	SALINE	IV	1000ml				8 hours		*A. Doctor # 123*								
2/2/15	DEXTROSE	IV	1000ml				8 hours		*A. Doctor # 123*								

Scenario 6

Please prescribe first-line acute treatment for a patient with serum potassium levels of 6.6 mmol/L, with tented T waves on his ECG. He is asymptomatic and has normal haemodynamic parameters.

ONCE ONLY MEDICINES

1. Patient away from ward   3. Patient refused does   5. Dose not given at nurse's discretion
2. Patient could not take dose   4. Dose not available   6. Dose not given at doctor's request
7. Self administration

Date Prescribed	Approved Name of Medicine	Date and Time Due	Dose	Route	Signature & Bleep No.	
2/2/15	CLACIUM GLUCONATE 109	1800,2/2/15	100mg	IV	[signature] A. Doctor #123	

RECORD OF INFUSION THERAPY

Date	Infusion fluid	Route	Volume of infusion	Additives Approved name	Additives Dose	Batch No.	Rate of infusion	Start time	Prescriber's signature & bleep No.	Pharmacy	Infusion started Time	Infusion started Vol.	Infusion started By	Infusion started Check	Batch No.	Pump No.	Reason not to administ.
2/2/15	DEXTROSE 50%	IV	50ml	INSULIN	10u		30 mins		✓ H. Doctor #123								

Scenario 7

A patient is admitted to the ED with an acute severe exacerbation of asthma. Please review this prescription for the initial doses of first-line medication.

OXYGEN	Device*	N=Nasal cannula SM = Simple face mask RM = Reservoir mask V = Venturi					
Date	2/2/15			**0600**	% or L/min		
Target Saturation %		94% — 98%			Device		
					Initials		
Humidified Y/N				**1200**	% or L/min		
% or L/min		Titrate to target saturation as per BTS guideline			Device		
Device*					Initials		
Duration/Time to titration				**1800**	% or L/min		
					Device		
Signature Print name bleep no.	*A. Doctor #123*	Initials	Initials		Initials		
				2200	% or L/min		
Administration started		Date	Time	Initials	Device		
					Initials		

Approved Name of Antibiotic	Dose	Freq	Pharmacist Check	Date / Time		
Signature Print name bleep no.	Start date	Route	Pharmacist Check			
	Duration					
Indication/Restricted code						

ONCE ONLY MEDICINES

1. Patient away from ward
2. Patient could not take dose
7. Self administration

3. Patient refused does
4. Dose not available

5. Dose not given at nurse's discretion
6. Dose not given at doctor's request

Date Prescribed	Approved Name of Medicine	Date and Time Due	Dose	Route	Signature & Bleep No.	
2/2/15	HYDROCORTISONE	STAT	100mg	ORAL	A. Doctor #123	
2/2/15	SALBUTAMOL	STAT	5 mcg	NEB	A. Doctor #123	

Scenario 8

Please review this prescription for an initial sliding scale for a type 1 diabetic with sepsis and uncontrolled blood glucose. She has been vomiting and is not eating or drinking. Her BM is currently 11 and her serum potassium is 4.0 mmol/L. Renal function is normal.

INTRAVENOUS INSULIN PRESCRIPTION – Insulin (human soluble) 50 units in 50 mls sodium chloride 0.9%

Start with standard insulin regimen. Check meter BG hourly and adjust insulin infusion rate accordingly.

Blood glucose (mmol/L)	Standard insulin Regime (units/hour)	Reduced Regime (units/hour)	Augmented Regime 1 (units/hour)	Augmented Regime 2 (units/hour)	Altered Regime 3 (units/hour)
0 – 3.9	0	0	0	0	
4 – 6.9	0.5	0	1	1	
7 – 8.9	1	0.5	2	2	
9 – 10.9	2	1	3	4	
11 – 13.9	3	2	4	6	
14 – 19.9	4	3	6	8	
≥ 20	6	4	9	12	
Start date, time and nurse's signature					
Discontinued date, time and nurse's signature					
Date, time, doctor's signature and bleep No.	A. Doctor #123				1800 2/2/15

RECORD OF INFUSION THERAPY

| Date | Infusion fluid | Route | Volume of infusion | Additives | | | Rate of infusion | Start time | Prescriber's signature & bleep No. | Pharmacy | Infusion started | | | | | Batch No. | Pump No. | Reason not to administ. |
				Approved name	Dose	Batch No.					Time	Vol.	By	Initials	Check			
2/2/15	DEXTROSE 10%	IV	500ml	KCl	20 mmol				A. Doctor #123									

ANSWERS

Scenario 1

REGULAR MEDICATION																	

Approved Name of Medicine		Dose		Freq	Time												
IBUPROFEN		400mg		TDS	⑧												
Additional instructions		Start date	Route														
FOR BACK PAIN		2/2/15	ORAL		⑭												
Signature	Pharmacist check	POD	Supply														
					㉒												
Print name	Bleep no.																
A. Doctor #123																	

Approved Name of Medicine		Dose		Freq	Time												
OMEPRAZOLE		20mg		OD													
Additional instructions FOR NSAID GASTRO PROCTECTION		Start date 2/2/15	Route ORAL		⑧												
Signature	Pharmacist check	POD	Supply														
Print name	Bleep no.																
A. Doctor #123																	

Approved Name of Medicine		Dose		Freq	Time												
Additional instructions		Start date	Route														
Signature	Pharmacist check	POD	Supply														
Print name	Bleep no.																

- PPIs are recommended as gastro-intestinal protection.
- The frequency of PPI administration has been omitted, OD should be included.
- In order to minimize the duration of NSAID therapy, the prescriber should also highlight that this medication should be reviewed regularly.

Scenario 2

OXYGEN	Device*	N=Nasal cannula SM = Simple face mask RM = Reservoir mask V = Venturi					
Date						0600	% or L/min	
Target Saturation %							Device	
							Initials	
Humidified Y/N		Titrate to target saturation as per BTS guideline				1200	% or L/min	
% or L/min							Device	
Device*							Initials	
Duration/Time to titration						1800	% or L/min	
							Device	
Signature Print name bleep no.			Initials	Initials			Initials	
						2200	% or L/min	
Administration started		Date	Time	Initials			Device	
							Initials	

Approved Name of Antibiotic	Dose	Freq	Pharmacist Check	Date / Time	2/2/15
DOXYCYCLINE	100mg	OD		⑧	✕
					SEE
Signature *[signature]* Print name bleep no. A. Doctor # 123	Start date 2/2/15	Route ORAL	Pharmacist Check		ONCE ONLY MEDS
	Duration 5/7				
Indication/Restricted code					

ONCE ONLY MEDICINES

1. Patient away from ward
2. Patient could not take dose
3. Patient refused does
4. Dose not available
5. Dose not given at nurse's discretion
6. Dose not given at doctor's request
7. Self administration

Date Prescribed	Approved Name of Medicine	Date and Time Due	Dose	Route	Signature & Bleep No.	
2/2/15	DOXYCYCLINE	1400, 2/2/15	200mg	ORAL	*Dr A. Doctor* #123	

- This indication requires a loading dose of 200 mg followed by regular dosing of 100 mg.
- Typically the loading dose would be prescribed on the 'stat' side, and the regular dose on the regular side (specific antibiotic prescriptions will be available at some trusts).
- Ensure that the dates are filled appropriately and the duration of therapy is indicated, usually in the 'additional instructions' box (typical total course duration is 5 days – written as 'total course 5/7', or 'to complete 5/7 course').

Scenario 3

AS REQUIRED MEDICATION												
Approved Name of Medicine ORAMORPH 10 mg/ 5 ml	Dose 10 mg	Route ORAL	Date									
Additional instructions	Min. interval 2 hourly	Max. in 24 hours 60mg	Time									
			Dose									
Signature [signature]	Start date 2/2/15	Pharmacist check	Route									
Print name A. Doctor # 123 Bleep no.	POD	Supply	Given									
Approved Name of Medicine	Dose	Route	Date									
Additional instructions	Min. interval	Max. in 24 hours	Time									
			Dose									
Signature	Start date	Pharmacist check	Route									
Print name Bleep no.	POD	Supply	Given									

- When prescribing liquids remember to state the concentration.
- For Oramorph this is typically 10 mg/5 mL (note 100 mg/5 mL solution exists). Ensure that the interval allows time for the dose to be effective and will not lead to overdose.
- Also ensure that the daily maximum is within an amount you consider appropriate for the patient (taking into account weight, renal function etc.).

Scenario 4

STH WARFARIN PRESCRIPTION AND MONITORING CHART

Indication for treatment ___DVT___	Name: *FRANCIS BACON*
Target INR range ___2·5 (RANGE 2-3)___ (see over)	DOB: 2/3/45
Recommended duration of treatment (please tick):	Hosp No.: *AB 1234*
6 weeks ☐ 12 weeks ☑ 6 months ☐ long term ☐	NHS No.:
Newly starting treatment? (please tick):	Ward Consultant
Yes ☑ No ☐ (usual dose ___ mg)	A1 *AAB*
INR monitored by: GP ☐ STH clinic ☐ other ☐ ___	

Chronic Atrial Fibrillation (without an established thromboembolic event)
Cross through the dosing chart overleaf and follow STH Warfarin Slow Start Regimen.
Elderly Patients
1. High risk of drug interaction with warfarin due to likelihood of higher co-morbidity and polypharmacy.
2. Decision to initiate should take into account likely compliance, attendance for INR checks and risk of falling.
3. Normal ageing and/or acute ill health may require treatment to be reviewed in light of point 2 above.
Cancer Patients
Patients with active malignancy, particularly if receiving chemo/radiotherapy, should be considered for ongoing treatment with low molecular weight heparin. Discuss with oncology consultant or ask for haematology advice.
Tromboembolic Disease in Pregnancy and the Puerperium
Avoid warfarin therapy during pregnancy. Seek advice from an obstetrician on heparin treatment in pregnancy and warfarin initiation in the puerperium.

MONITORING AND DOSING GUIDANCE OVERLEAF

WARFARIN if baseline INR is greater than 1.4 seek advice from the responsible consultant.
the prescribing doctor must know the baseline INR before signing the first dose of warfarin.

Date	INR	Oral dose in milligrams (to be given at 6p)m	Signature of prescriber	Signature of administering nurse
2/2/15	Baseline 1.0	10 mg	*A. Doctor#123*	

- Ensure baseline INR is documented and is in the appropriate range for warfarin administration at appropriate dose.
- Highlighting the INR box for the following day indicates that an INR must be recorded prior to further warfarin dose prescription.
- Regarding duration of therapy, consider if reversible factors are present. If in doubt consult a senior colleague (see Ch. 14).

Scenario 5

RECORD OF INFUSION THERAPY

Date	Infusion fluid	Route	Volume of infusion	Additives Approved name	Additives Dose	Batch No.	Rate of infusion	Start time	Prescriber's signature & bleep No.	Pharmacy	Infusion started Time	Vol.	Initials By	Initials Check	Batch No.	Pump No.	Reason not to administ.
2/2/15	DEXTROSE 5%	IV	1000ml	POTASSIUM CHORIDE	20 mmol		8 hours		*signature* H. Doctor #123								
2/2/15	SALINE 0.9%	IV	1000ml	POTASSIUM CHORIDE	20 mmol		8 hours		*signature* H. Doctor #123								
2/2/15	DEXTROSE 5%	IV	1000ml	POTASSIUM CHORIDE	20 mmol		8 hours		*signature* H. Doctor #123								

- Fluids prescription must always take into account multiple patient factors, including daily requirements for electrolytes (see Ch. 15, Section 15.1).
- Maintenance fluids should usually contain around 2 mmol/kg sodium and 1 mmol/kg potassium per 24 hours. Each bag should therefore have 20 mmol potassium added.
- The % value of the fluids should be stated.
- For further advice and alternatives see Chapter 15.

Scenario 6

ONCE ONLY MEDICINES		
1. Patient away from ward	3. Patient refused does	5. Dose not given at nurse's discretion
2. Patient could not take dose	4. Dose not available	6. Dose not given at doctor's request
7. Self administration		

Date Prescribed	Approved Name of Medicine	Date and Time Due	Dose	Route	Signature & Bleep No.	
2/2/15	CALCIUM GLUCONATE 10%	1800, 2/2/15	10 m/s	IV	*[signature]* A. Doctor #123	

- Calcium gluconate concentration not included (should read calcium gluconate 10%).
  - May be repeated every 10 minutes until ECG normalizes.
  - Consider additional prescription of salbutamol nebulizer.
- Insulin should normally be prescribed by brand name to avoid confusion (for IV, Actrapid® is frequently used).
- When prescribing insulin, always write 'Units' (not U or IU).
- Ensure potassium is checked 2 hours after insulin administration (see Ch. 15, Section 15.1).

Scenario 7

OXYGEN		Device*	N=Nasal cannula SM = Simple face mask RM = Reservoir mask V = Venturi						
Date	2/2/15				**0600**	% or L/min			
Target Saturation %		94% 88%				Device			
						Initials			
Humidified Y/N	N					% or L/min			
% or L/min	15L	Titrate to target saturation as per BTS guideline			**1200**	Device			
Device*	NON RE BREAHE					Initials			
Duration/Time to titration					**1800**	% or L/min			
						Device			
Signature _A Doctr_ Print name bleep no. _A. Doctor #123_			Initials	Initials		Initials			
Administration started			Date	Time	Initials	**2200**	% or L/min		
						Device			
						Initials			

Approved Name of Antibiotic	Dose	Freq	Pharmacist Check	Date / Time		
Signature Print name bleep no.	Start date	Route	Pharmacist Check			
	Duration					
Indication/Restricted code						

ONCE ONLY MEDICINES

1. Patient away from ward   3. Patient refused does   5. Dose not given at nurse's discretion
2. Patient could not take dose   4. Dose not available   6. Dose not given at doctor's request
7. Self administration

Date Prescribed	Approved Name of Medicine	Date and Time Due	Dose	Route	Signature & Bleep No.	
2/2/15	HYDROCORTISON	2/2/15,1900	100mg	IV	*Dott* A. Doctor #123	
2/2/15	SALBUTAMOL	2/2/15,1900	5mg	NEB	*Dott* A. Doctor #123	

- Oxygen is a drug and therefore should be prescribed (prescription type will vary by trust).
- If a specific oxygen delivery system is required it should be stated (e.g. nasal cannula, non-rebreathe mask) and reviewed as appropriate to maintain saturations >94%.
- STAT is not appropriate terminology for timing of once only medications. The time and date should be documented to aid later analysis of prescription and to indicate the time between prescription and administration.
- Hydrocortisone is administered IV for asthma (oral prednisolone 40 mg is an acceptable alternative to hydrocortisone 100 mg IV QDS in a patient able to swallow).
- Salbutamol nebulised dose is 5 mg (not mcg – which should be written in full as micrograms when used, to reduce the risk of dosing errors). A smaller dose (2.5 mg) may also be used and has less risk of tachycardia.

Scenario 8

INTRAVENOUS INSULIN PRESCRIPTION – Insulin (human soluble) 50 units in 50 mls sodium chloride 0.9%					
Start with standard insulin regimen. Check meter BG hourly and adjust insulin infusion rate accordintly.					
Blood glucose (mmol/L)	Standard insulin Regime (units/hour)	Reduced Regime (units/hour)	Augmented Regime 1 (units/hour)	Augmented Regime 2 (units/hour)	Altered Regime 3 (units/hour)
0 – 3.9	0	0	0	0	
4 – 6.9	0.5	0	1	1	
7 – 8.9	1	0.5	2	2	
9 – 10.9	2	1	3	4	
11 – 13.9	3	2	4	6	
14 – 19.9	4	3	6	8	
≥ 20	6	4	9	12	
Start date, time and nurse's signature					
Discontinued date, time and nurse's signature					
Date, time, doctor's signature and bleep No.	*Date* A. Doctor # 123				

Self-assessment

RECORD OF INFUSION THERAPY

Date	Infusion fluid	Route	Volume of infusion	Additives			Rate of infusion	Start time	Prescriber's signature & bleep No.	Pharmacy	Infusion started					Batch No.	Pump No.	Reason not to administ.
				Approved name	Dose	Batch No.					Time	Vol.	Initials					
													By	Check				
2/2/15	DEXTROSE 10% (for sliding scale when BM 2 w)	IV	500ml	POTASSIUM CHLORIDE	20 mmol		50 ml/hr		*sig* A. Doctor #123									
	(Alternative insulin prescription for sliding scale)																	
2/2/15	SODIUM CHLORIDE 0.9%	IV	50ml	HUMAN SOLUBLE INSULIN	50 UNITS		AS PER PROTOCOL		*sig* A. Doctor #123									

The figure given above shows an example of a sliding scale regimen.

- A proforma may not be available in all settings and in this case the insulin should be prescribed with the infusion therapy.
  - Prescribe in record of infusion therapy: sodium chloride 0.9% 50 mL with 50 units soluble human insulin (or Actrapid), rate – as per protocol. (See alternative insulin prescription described in the figure above.)
- NB: The protocol will additionally need to be prescribed either on the kardex or in the notes (as per local protocol). The proforma sliding scale shown may be used as a guide for this prescription.
- Glucose infusions must run alongside insulin where blood glucose is not significantly raised (>14 mmol/L or as per local policy), and run at 50 mL/h.
- Potassium should be added where serum levels are not raised (often <5 mmol/L), but should be written as potassium chloride and not prescribed as the molecular formula.
- Additional fluids may be prescribed for either fluid maintenance/resuscitation as appropriate (see Ch. 16, Section 16.1).

Index